Doctorin' Oil Field Trash:
True Tales of Roughnecks & Rougher Women from Spindletop to Saratoga

G. P. Stoker, M.D.

Edited by Michelle M. Haas

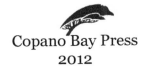

Copano Bay Press
2012

Originally published in 1948 under the title *Oil Field Medico*

ISBN 978-0-9884357-0-4

TABLE OF CONTENTS

Publisher's Note

The surreal landscapes that were the early Texas oil fields, with derrick after derrick standing dutifully at attention as far as the eye could see, were bound to breed an even more surreal species of inhabitants in the accompanying boom-towns. The combination of money, life-threatening work and fearless folks with pioneering spirits created a carnival-like atmosphere the likes of which most of us can scarcely imagine. Dr. Stoker's memoirs give us a concrete understanding of the madness that reigned at places like Spindletop and Batson Prairie at the turn of the last century, preserving for future generations a sense of life in the early Texas fields.

Michelle M. Haas, Managing Editor
Seven Palms - Rockport, TX

Texas' First Oil Gusher

A slow drizzling rain was falling as I stepped out of the Pullman and took my bag from the porter's hand. A narrow, muddy street ran in front of the station. Men in high boots were swinging and cracking long whips over the backs of mule teams. The teams were wallowing in mud up to their bellies, straining to pull the wagons laden with heavy pipe and other oil well supplies, plunging, falling into the mud, getting up to lunge again, as the singing whips tore at their backs, and the raw curses of the mule-skinners filled the air. A wave of distaste and excitement swept over me as I viewed the scene. I had left my growing practice of medicine with all its bright prospects for the very thing I was looking at. I set out with high heart on this adventure, lured by the thrilling tales of the Croesus-like fortunes being made in the black gold flowing from Texas' first oil gushers. I decided that no fastidiousness of mine should cause me to turn back, at least until I had seen whether or not what I had heard was true.

Before arriving in Beaumont, I had been told that the Crosby was the best hotel in town. In answer to my inquiries of its whereabouts, the station agent laconically pointed across the street. There it stood like an old scow pushed up against the banks of a river. I gingerly picked my way through the mud to the uninteresting, ramshackle, one-story frame building with an apparent afterthought of an extra story in the rear. The lower story, one room wide, running out like an extended invitation, had a roof as steep and pointed as an Alpine mountaineer's hat. Around the entrance ran a wide gallery which had been divided into narrow stall-like places by planks nailed to the wall of the building and the bannister of the gallery. Over the unfinished boards of the walls were tacked blueprints of the Great Spindle-Top Oil Field. Tables and crude homemade desks were covered with maps showing future locations for derricks on the leases. Men who had rented these stalls as offices were selling locations as fast as they could sign the papers and receive the money.

An intense air of excitement pervaded the place. Men and women, gesticulating wildly, ran from one stall to another. Stacks of green-backs stood out in vivid contrast against the blue of the maps. I had never seen so much money. I stood and watched with amazement as hundreds of thousands of dollars were exchanged for future oil wells in the Great Spindle-Top Oil Field, Texas' first gusher field.

As my bag became heavy in my hand, I realized that I had not yet obtained a room at the hotel. So I crossed the narrow place boarded off on the gallery and entered the hotel lobby. A roar of noise burst upon my ears. The high-pitched, strained voices of women, mingled with the coarser voices of men; oaths and curses exploded through a haze of cigarette, cigar, and pipe smoke which hung over the lobby. A milling throng of humanity of every type moved in groups or alone. Well-dressed, prosperous businessmen stood talking to the rough-neck in high boot and slicker suit. Disheveled, hardfaced women screamed at each other above the din. The one theme of all was oil leases.

I stepped up to the desk, made of rough planks nailed together and painted a bilious-looking brown. A sallow-faced clerk, his dark hair plastered back from his narrow forehead, looked at me with bored, indifferent eyes. I told him I should like to engage a room, but he informed me all rooms were occupied. When I asked him if he did not have a cot he might give me to sleep on in a hall, he grew a bit more eloquent and informed me that all space in the halls was at present occupied with cots. Then waving his hand toward the uncomfortable-looking chairs in the lobby, he told me he could not even give me a seat, for they had all been rented for months every night. Not because of lack of money, he said; for the people who occupied those chairs in the lobby at night often carried in their pockets a hundred thousand dollars in currency. That left me in an uncertain mood.

I had come to Beaumont with the idea of perhaps locating and practicing medicine in the oil field. But I had never heard of or met conditions such as were being described to me. I asked the clerk what prospects for hotel accommodations existed out at Spindle-Top. He said that everyone who could, came into Beaumont at night, but if I wanted to go out and see for myself, I could take a hack and drive out to the field. Something in his tone caused my mood to become more uncertain of any comfortable place in Spindle-Top. And, he continued, he did not think I would have much choice as to hacks, for they were all about alike. The important thing was to get one with horses that could get through the mud.

My introduction to the oil field was diverting, to say the least; just off the train, no room to sleep in, on all sides of me persons, to all appearances, lunatics, who could chatter about only one thing, and that one thing, oil. Since I was here, I thought, I might as well see the place which was causing these people to go so crazy. I picked up my bag, which was getting to be a nuisance, went out of the lobby and down to the street corner where a motley array of horses, hacks and drivers stood. It looked to me as if neither hackman, hack, nor horse could go through much of anything, certainly not deep, sticky mud. Finally I came to one driver who assured me he could make the trip in nothing flat, or better. His old gray and black horses did not look encouraging but I thought with proper persuasion they might possibly make it. So I engaged him and his outfit, climbed in the hack and sat down on a lumpy, sagging, springless seat. The "hackie" hit the ribs of the horses a sharp tap, and with a lurch which nearly threw me out of the seat, we were off.

Down the street we galloped, mud and water making merry with the passersby, until the burst of speed that each crack of the whip put into the sad-looking nags exhausted itself, and we settled down to a more prudent pace. The streets were checker-boards of mud and deep holes, made by the wagons carrying pipe and heavy machinery for the oil field. These holes were filled with water. If the horses made a misstep into one of these, the old hack would lurch and list from side to side, as if it were on a stormy sea. But the "hackie" told me to hold to my seat and assured me that we would neither flounder nor sink. The rough sailing was made more bearable by the beauty of the stately magnolias and cape-jasmine trees, which lined the mud holes that Beaumont called streets. These extended to the edge of the city.

We finally encountered the old shell road which ran through the flat, dreary looking saltgrass-covered land. This road had been graded up several feet and covered with shell, so the wagons hauling the heavy oil-field machinery would not sink down out of sight into the mud holes. Sometimes there would be a stretch of fifty yards without a mud hole, and again, the horses would strain through a slippery, sliding mass of water and mud, almost up to their bellies. The rain which had not abated since I stepped off the train, drifted down over the black marshy ground which had only an occasional scrubby-looking tree to break the flatness of the scene. And as steady as the rain, so was the "hackie's" continual stream of oil field history. He paused only when he shifted his cud of tobacco from one side of his jaw to the other, or when, he tried to overflow a mud hole with a stream of tobacco juice as he discharged it with amazing accuracy at some object in the road.

In place of the magnolia trees of Beaumont, saloons now lined the road. The "hackie" knew the names of the owners and bartenders of each. Suddenly the first oil derrick came into sight. The loquacious driver gave me its history, the name of each member of the company who owned it and of the contractor who had drilled it. As we rode on, derricks became more numerous. By the time we entered the main part of the Spindle-Top oil field, we were driving down a lane of derricks with just enough room between them for two vehicles to pass each other. As we approached the business section of Spindle-Top, the "hackie" asked me where I wanted to go. I did not answer his question, for by now my burning desire was to catch a train out of that mud hole and go back home. Instead I suggested that he take me to the best hotel in town. He turned around in his seat and looked at me with a surprised stare.

Spraying tobacco juice over the street he drawled, "There ain't no best hotel, but there's a place yuh kin stay if yuh wanna, that is if they ain't full up."

By this time we were going down the muddy road of the main street of Spindle-Top. Crazy-looking shacks leered down at me from the stilts they sat upon. Mud, water and oil made small pools under them. The driver stopped at one of these, which was a little larger than the others, and said, "Well, Kid, here yuh air."

I paid him, took my bag, and stepped down. A fountain of mud, oil, and water burst forth to greet my shoes and the lower part of my pants. Two jumps and I landed on a boardwalk in front of the larger shack. From its sign I knew it was a hotel. My pants and shoes were dripping a black, greasy substance, mud and water mixed with Spindle-Top oil, which was not only in the air, but also on the ground. Mud and water was sloshing in my socks as I walked and words were sloshing in my mind about Spindle-Top and her streets. I glanced up from my mud-laden legs and there, in that mire which was called a street, were men, up to their knees in the mud and water, driving mule and ox-teams carrying heavy machinery which sank the wheels down to their hubs. Some of the men were laughing, others singing and some were swearing. I felt like joining the last group. I cleaned my shoes and the bottom of my trousers a bit with my handkerchief, picked up my bag, which had accompanied me through university, medical school and travels, and walked into the hotel.

I INHERIT A PRACTICE

Unpainted, twelve-inch planks formed the walls, ceiling, and floors of the hotel. Mud had made a carpet on the floor, where a carpet should have been. Half-drunken people filled the lobby. The same atmosphere of wild excitement and the same theme—oil—as in Beaumont, met me as I entered the place. I walked over to the desk, which was made of rough unpainted plank, and asked the clerk for a room. He called a tough-looking Negro, garbed in dirty clothes, to take my bag and show me to my room. Down a narrow corridor we went to the end of the hall. He opened the door, set my bag in, gave me the key and, after I had tipped him, left me. I closed the door and looked around. A musty, damp smell pervaded the room. It was small and bare, made out of the same unpainted lumber as the lobby. A half-sized, sagging bed covered with dirty linen, which had been used by many former guests without recourse to the laundry, stood in one corner. Through an unwashed window which could boast only a few cobwebs for a curtain, streamed the gray light. A broken mirror hung over the washstand on which stood a bowl with a dark-looking rim, a mute reminder of the previous washings of many oily hands. A used, dirty towel was thrown in a discouraged way over the stained water pitcher. One broken chair leaned rakishly against the wall. I went over to the small table on which were a small pitcher and an unwashed tumbler. The pitcher was filled with water.

Being thirsty, I poured out a glass of water and raised it to my lips. One swallow and I set the glass down. If that was Spindle-Top's drinking water, I knew why I had seen so many drunken men in the hotel lobby!

I went back into the lobby. The people were streaming toward a large room. Its wide-open doors revealed a long table covered with dishes. I knew it was the dining room. And as my stomach was signaling to me that it needed food, I followed the crowd into the room and took a seat on one of the backless benches which stood on each side of the table. The table cloth may have been white when it was first bought, but too many greasy sleeves leaning on it to support the weight of the food on the owners' knives or forks had left the whiteness a dingy gray, with odd patterns of coffee stain, polka dots of egg yolk and gray splashes of gravy. Thick, white, cracked platters held half-cooked beans and a mass of smeary rice. Soggy, water-logged potatoes winked slyly at one with eyes which the cook had forgotten to remove. And what appeared to be steak floated in a weak looking gravy, adorned with chunks of grease.

I ate my dinner in silence, for my stomach was saying things to me about the type of food I was sending down to it. The table hummed with conversation about oil wells, fights, gambling, and women. I finished quickly and walked out on the street.

Some of the houses were sitting up on higher stilts than others. According to the height of the stilts of the shacks, one would have to step up or down on the boardwalk, which was a twelve-inch plank placed above and across the oily mud. With much care to keep my balance on this walk, I reached the corner and decided to cross the street. I was trying to choose the patch of mud which was less deep, when I saw two women start across the street. I waited to see what they would do. They stepped down and with short hops tried to make it to some oil-covered, half-submerged rocks in the road. Occasionally they slipped off the rocks and slid into the muddy water. Then the gray, drizzling rain would be pierced by electric oaths. After they were safely across, I tried their method and the same thing happened to me.

In this way successfully navigating two or three streets, I came to a shack on which was nailed a rough, four-inch board with a doctor's name painted on it. With dismay I saw that the outside of the house was as dreary and unkempt as the adjoining shacks. I stood and looked at it a moment and thought. Perhaps if I went in and talked to the doctor I might learn something to restore my courage. At least, I would be able to find a point of contact with another human being.

As I stood looking at the dreary scene, memories of the home of wealth in which I had been born and reared came to me. My father had sent me to the University where I became captain of both the baseball and football teams. After being graduated in medicine at a well-known medical college, I had opened up an office in my home town.

The art of baseball and football has changed much since I played it in those days. It took an iron man to go against the punishment of the opposing team. All things were allowed and football soon was attracting the attention of the world of sports as a murderous game, and a murderous game it was. Little did I know during those days at the University that my learning to take care of myself in tough places on the field would stand me in good stead in the oil field. Often I had heard the captain of an opposing team raise his head and call out to his players across the scrimmage line that he would give ten dollars to the man who would kill that red-headed quarterback. As I looked at the dirty, unkempt office of the doctor of the town I thought of the football field and wondered how I had made such a fumble that would penalize me into such a position from which to start the practice of medicine.

I walked up the broken steps, opened a door which led into the shack, and entered a small room which, evidently, was the waiting room. The walls were crude, unpainted, unpapered planks. One little dirty window and the cracks between the planks let in the light. A small, unpainted table in the center of the room and a few old chairs standing around the sides constituted the furniture. Not a very ritzy looking affair, I thought. While I was trying to make up my mind whether to leave or call the doctor, the door to the inner office opened, and a man about fifty-five years old stepped out. He was of medium height, with heavy, pouched eyes set in a dissipated face. Thick, gray, oily-looking hair stood up around his head. A crooked scar crossed his right cheek and stopped at a tobacco-stained moustache. His clothes were spotted and unpressed, his linen soiled and frayed. Looking me over slowly, he finally said, "What do you want?"

I gave him my name, told him I was a physician who had just arrived in town with the idea of opening an office and asked him if I could see the doctor. As I talked, I could see that he was trying to concentrate. When I finished speaking, he still remained in an attitude of thought. I did not interrupt him, and presently he opened his mouth. I tried to cover my dismay when he told me in a thick voice that *he* was the doctor.

A machine-gun spray of questions about myself followed. He wanted my history. I told him of myself, my days at the University and medical school, travel, experience in the practice of medicine and about my family. When I ended he said, "I believe you are the very damned guy I am looking for. I haven't been on a good drunk for six months. I am just on my way to see a patient. Come along with me, for I want to talk more to you."

I was so desperate from the dismal drip of the rain and from looking at the dirty, oily mud that I was delighted with the invitation. We walked down the street and, from the few words spoken, I began to realize there were doctors and *doctors*. Fresh from post-graduate work and a practice among a cultured university group, I had much to learn. We stopped in front of a shack and went in. The room in which I found myself was almost bare of furniture. The only light came through the cracks of the planks which made the house and through the door which stood ajar. There was no window in the room. As my eyes became accustomed to the darkness, I made out the form of a man lying on a cot. A dirty, stained comfort served him as a mattress. A torn, dirtier blanket covered his long-unwashed clothes. The doctor spoke to him, but the patient seemed too ill to answer clearly. Turning to me, he said, "Examine the patient, Doctor."

I leaned over and took the thin wrist in my hand. The pulse was irregular and weak. His skin felt dry, and he was burning with fever. I examined him and decided the patient was fatally ill with malaria and complications. When I had finished, the doctor rose and we stepped outside.

"What is the matter with him?" he asked me as we stood on the broken steps of the shack.

"All that ails him, Doctor, is that he is going to die unless he has hospital care at once, is my opinion," I replied.

"What would you do?" he asked me.

"Have you a hospital you can send him to?"

I had been taught in medical school that when a patient is going to die, I should send for another doctor or get him to a hospital so that the responsibility would not rest entirely on the attending physician's shoulders.

He stopped and looked at me as though that was the most intelligent thing I had said. Then he slapped me on the shoulder and said he could send the patient to the Catholic Sisters' Hospital at Beaumont. And best of all, he would go with the patient. We went back into the house and he told the patient that he was going to send for the ambulance from Beaumont at once, and that he himself would take him to the hospital. The patient muttered something that I did not understand, and the doctor and I went back to his office.

He invited me into his inner office for a little conversation. Turning to me as we sat down, he said, "I shall get the ambulance out here at once and take the patient to Beaumont. I want to go on a drunk, and I want you to stay here in my office, take my instruments, and care for my practice until I get back. What do you say?"

I was a bit startled and not very enthusiastic. As he saw me hesitate he continued, "You will have lots of work and make lots of money. I shall leave the patient at the hospital, and then I will go and get on a real drunk. I do not know when I will be back. But you take care of the office and patients and take the money and, when I get back, I'll take over again."

Before I could accept or refuse his offer, he was busy preparing to leave at once, his face wreathed in anticipatory smiles. I could almost hear him saying to himself, "What, oh, what a drunk I'll soon be on!"

As he went about packing a dilapidated bag, I turned his offer over in my mind. I had come to the oil fields with the idea of practicing my profession, and it seemed as though Lady Luck had stopped on my number with no effort on my part. So, I decided to accept the offer. Thus I inherited an office and a practice all within a few hours after I arrived at Spindle-Top.

The ambulance arrived. I helped to put the patient into it, the doctor climbed up on the seat with the driver, and they were off. From a description of the trip given me later by the driver of the ambulance, the doctor and he managed to get by the first saloon on the road to Beaumont. But the doctor saw no reason to waste time in starting on his drunk. By the time they arrived at the second saloon, he had sold the driver on the idea of taking one little drink. The rain had cleared away and a hot broiling sun shone down on the mud. The patient lay in the ambulance too sick to care that heat and steam from the wet earth enveloped him. The doctor and ambulance driver took their drink and drove on. They skipped the third saloon and stopped at the fourth, for by that time they were both very dry again. It took several drinks in that saloon to give them strength for their journey. They went on a few blocks and another saloon was standing there to invite them to enter and cool their burning throats. Each time they stopped they stayed longer, for their thirst increased the nearer they got to Beaumont.

Finally, sometime near midnight, they arrived in Beaumont. By that time it made no difference to the patient whether they stopped at the hospital or took him directly to the undertaker's establishment; for that was where he belonged.

I Meet Spindle-Top Patients

After the ambulance left with the doctor and his patient, I went through the bleak, dirty waiting room into the private office. In a small wooden box were his instruments—old, dirty, and stained. A shabby ancient operating-table stood near a rain-streaked, fly-specked window. Underneath the table the floor was littered with blood-stained cotton swabs. A bottle, partially filled with alcohol, stood on a plank, which he had evidently used as a service-table for his instruments when operating. I wondered whether or not alcohol had been used outside for sterilizing the instruments, or internally by the doctor.

I thought of my own well-equipped offices at home, the laboratory at the University with its X-ray and microscope where, until a few days before, I had been assistant to the Chair of Science and Research. The contrast between what I had left and what I had come into made me wonder whether or not I was having a bad dream. As I stood there thinking of what I had done, I heard a noise in the waiting room. Two men were entering, carrying a third between them. I saw that the left leg of his trousers had been torn away above the knee and an old dirty handkerchief now oozing blood had been wrapped around the leg.

They came into the inner office, put the man down on the dirty operating table, and asked for the doctor. I told them that he had just left for Beaumont with a patient.

"When in hell will he be back?" one of them roared.

"I don't know," I replied.

A stream of curses poured from their lips. Tiring at last, they stopped long enough to ask me whether the old son-of-a-bitch had left any one in charge of his office.

"I am the doctor he left in charge," I answered. A look of surprise passed over their faces.

"Sonny, don't tell us you're a doctor. Why, you're just a damn kid," one of them said.

I had been able to complete my medical studies in less than the prescribed time, and many times before this experience

I had found my youthful appearance was an obstacle I had to overcome.

"I am the doctor here. Will you kindly tell me what it is you want?" I said, trying to impress upon their minds the dignity of my profession.

"Well, I'll be dammed," muttered one, "maybe the kid is a doctor."

"Aw, hell! Stop beefin'. John's gotta have help," growled the other. And turning to me he continued, "Kid, take a look at that son-of-a-bitch's leg. He just got the damn thing tore open out in the field. Can you fix it?"

I crossed over to the injured man and untied the dirty blood-soaked handkerchief from his leg. Blood spurted like a small geyser from a severed artery. Rummaging in the little wooden box, I discovered bandages, needles, thread, and makeshifts enough to stop the hemorrhage which was threatening the man's life. Washing and sterilizing my hands and the instruments, to the evident amazement of my spectators, I went to work on the injured leg. I soon had the wound sewed up and dressed. Turning to the interested man, I said, "You can take him to his home now, but I shall have to see him for a few days."

"Well, I'll, be damned, Kid, yuh did that quicker'n better'n the old man. Who the hell are yuh? Where'd yuh come from?" both of them began asking at once.

"I came here to stay," was all I answered. "Tell me where I can see the patient tomorrow."

Giving me the man's address, the speaker reached a dirty hand into the pockets of his oil-spotted trousers and handed me a twenty dollar bill.

"You'll do," he laughed. "Here's your pay for this work. We'll take this guy to his house. Yuh take care o' him till he gets well. We'll pay yuh."

It was well that they were busy picking up the injured man and did not see the surprise on my face. Twenty dollars for an office call was not what I had been in the habit of receiving. Just starting in the practice of medicine in a new town with a twenty dollar office fee in my pocket made the dirty office and muddy street seem much cleaner and brighter. How often the possession of money changes the outlook on this old mud-ball!

After they left, I turned and started to clean the old instruments and the office. By nightfall the place had taken on a different appearance.

Closing the office, I went back to the hotel. On the way I passed by the main drug store of the town and decided to go in and introduce myself. Word had spread over town during the afternoon that the old doctor had gone to Beaumont and had left a "kid-doctor" in his office.

When I introduced myself to the druggist, several field-workers and drillers were in the drug store. I knew from the way they stopped their conversation that I had been it subject.

The continuous rain, the mud and oil must have dampened all enthusiasm the druggist ever had. He did not seem to care whether or not if I was too young or the old doctor had really left. I talked with the drillers in the drug store awhile, but they were more interested in the oil-field, gambling, and fighting than in old or new doctors. They informed me that the doctor was a damned old drunken bastard and didn't know any medicine, but he did the best he could.

I went to the hotel, ate another dubious dinner and drifted out to see the town. The streets were thronged with drillers, rough-necks, business men, and prostitutes. As I walked down the street, I noticed that there was scarcely a store, gambling house, or saloon that had a door, and that almost every gambling house had its own saloon under the same roof. They did not need doors for business people were on a twenty-four hour shift, ladies and all.

The gambling house that I first entered had its saloon in the front of the place. It was ablaze with light. Pimps, professional gamblers, drillers, gun-men and business men stood at the bar, drinking, arguing, swearing and telling filthy stories. I went back to the gambling room which was thronged with all classes of people. Games were being played by tense, excited men. Cold-eyed, expressionless attendants of the games sat behind the tables pushing forward money or chips, or putting into the drawers the losings of the players. Earnings of a week were tossed on a number or a roll of the dice and lost. The betting ran high. Stacks of currency, piles of gold and silver stood in front of the eager-eyed players. Numbers were droned. The click of dice, the whirl of the wheel, wild laughter, and oaths filled the air. Half-dressed prostitutes stood with their arms around drunken men, sat in their laps or danced with them in vulgar postures. Men cursed them or pushed them away, if their overtures interrupted what they were doing. Old, haggard creatures with dyed hair, sensuous lips, and painted, wrinkled faces mingled with pretty young girls whose freshness had not yet hardened into a look of lust and greed.

The news had spread that the old doctor, who was a frequenter of these places, had gone to get on a drunk, and that a damned "kid" doctor had taken his place. Curious stares met me as I went from one gambling place to another. All were filled with the same class of people doing the same thing. "Old hags," many of whom had seen many winters before I was born, would call out to me, "Hello, Kid, buy me a drink," or "Say, Kid, ain't you going to take me for your sweetie?" Their invitations had no appeal to me and, after visiting a number of the places, I returned to my room in the hotel. My mind was whirling with mingled revolt and fascination for this strange life in the Spindle-Top oil field.

The next morning I arose early and, after breakfast, went to the office. The rain was coming down in sheets. The throngs of the night before had deserted the streets, and a lonely, gray, dirty, dreary place it was. Mules and ox teams floundered in the mud, straining to pull the heavy machinery out to the derricks, as lurid oaths fell from the lips of their drivers. I walked on to the office and had just opened the door when a call came to go out to the oil field to see a sick baby.

I found the family living in a tent which was surrounded by mud, water, and a few rocks. Pieces of half-submerged boards kept one from sinking into the mire up to his knees.

The tent had a dirt floor. Three half-ragged, tow-headed children, with sores on their faces, played listlessly in a corner. The baby lay in a large box which had contained dry goods before it had graduated to the status of a baby's bed. I found the baby a small, thin, yellow-faced thing with a well-developed case of rickets. I prescribed for it, and I saw the mother's dull-blue eyes and knew that she barely grasped the instructions I left with her. As I returned to my office, I thought that since I had been in Spindle-Top I had seen only dirt, sickness, squalor and the lowest form of sin.

When I entered my office, a call was waiting for me to go to another part of the field to an accident case. When I arrived at the scene of the accident, I found a man on a derrick floor almost torn to pieces. He was bleeding from the head, arm, and leg. After I had examined him, I did not know what to do with him. I knew I could not move him, and I felt it was dangerous to attempt to do anything for him under these insanitary conditions. As there was no other alternative, I decided to take a chance and patch him up. I told the boss of the rig that I wanted to give the patient an anaesthetic.

The suffering man heard me and said, "Hell, no, Doc, just give me a big drink of whiskey and go ahead." Before I could protest, one of the drillers standing near handed him a bottle almost filled with whiskey. He took the bottle in his uninjured hand, lifted it and said, "Here's to the bottom if it's a mile," put it to his lips and, when he handed the bottle back, it was empty. Looking up at me, he said, "Let's go, Doc."

The boss had them bring me hot water from the boiler and told me that if I needed anything to let him know. Leaving one man to assist me, he hurried the other men back on the job and started drilling again.

The man proved to be a good patient and as I worked with him I could not help admiring his iron nerves. Blood was spurting from a severed artery, and his arm was broken in several places. I stopped the blood, but I discovered that I had no splints with me. Noticing some pieces of board lying on the floor, I had my helper make me some temporary ones so that I might set his broken arm. When I had finally finished with him, I asked the boss of the rig to fix up a rude stretcher, and we sent the patient to his home. As I started back to the office the boss called to me and said, "Doc, you are new here. Have you ever seen an oil field before?" When he learned of the little I knew about an oil field, he offered to walk back with me to my office and take me through the main part of the famous Spindle-Top oil field.

As we passed among the derricks which were built closer together than in any other oil field in the world, I saw them touching and overlapping each other, often with one corner of a derrick inside another, the floor having been cut away to give room. All was feverish excitement. Wagons jostled each other as they crowded for room. Mules plunged and reared, ox teams pulled back. Men cursed and lashed their animals, while others almost came to blows with each other trying to maneuver for positions where they would have room enough to unload their pipe or machinery. The boss said, "We'll go down where they are expecting to bring in a well any minute. The drill is just about to the level where they will strike the oil. They have a strong gas pressure so they should get a gusher."

Just before we reached it, I saw the men working around the well fly into action at great speed. The boss said to me, "She's coming." Then we heard a bubbling, hissing noise, and I saw a six-inch stream of black oil spout up into the air hundreds of feet above the derrick with a roaring, blowing sound. As the oil shot above the derrick, the wind which was blowing from the south caused the oil to fall in a spray to the north covering all nearby houses, derricks, tanks, and the ground with the black liquid as the crew worked frantically to save it by directing it into a nearby earthen tank.

I found myself thrilling with excitement as I watched the black gold roar from the earth. I turned to look at the workmen and spectators and found, to my surprise, that to them it seemed a very ordinary event. No one thought it anything for a six-inch stream of oil to shoot up more than a hundred feet above the ground with no power save the gas pressure from the depths of the earth which forced it into the air. I was so fascinated that I stood and gazed spell-bound until my companion said, "Come on, Doc, you will get used to such sights as this." He was right, for I soon saw Saratoga, Batson Prairie, Sour Lake, and Humble bring in their wells to make the name of Texas world famous as a producer of liquid gold.

I Shoot Dice With A New Papa

I had been in the oil field some weeks. People continued to pour into the region, and the oil madness increased rather than abated. A strange, tense excitement prevailed and held all of us in its grasp. The revulsion which I felt during the first few days of my stay in Spindle-Top passed. The incredible brutality, the gross and flagrant bestiality, the crass ignorance of the people, the loss of life through lack of sanitation, indifference, and violence made me mentally nauseated at first. But the intangible, sinister, and hypnotic wildness dominated and submerged all things, and I soon found myself rushing through the days as wildly as the others.

Day by day my medical work increased until I was going almost constantly day and night. Often, in order to get a bit of sleep, I would have the hotel man tell the people who came for me that I was not there. But if I heard anyone say "Doctor," I was wide awake and up and going again. I forced my overtaxed body and nerves to respond to the hysterical urge about me, and was thrilled over the money piling up to my credit in the flimsy bank. My work consisted of everything, from treating a toothache, to laying down the pulseless hand of a person called by sudden death from too much whiskey, pistol shots, or a fight.

The habitues of the saloons, gambling houses, and the places where ladies of "easy morals" lived, were always sick, or in need of patching up after an argument which could not be settled in peace. I used to be called to these places to attend the girls, sometimes to find one of them dying from having drunk carbolic acid or some other kind of poison.

Many of these unfortunate women were young and beautiful, but it did not take long to destroy all semblance of beauty in that place of degradation. Once they entered that life, it seemed all hope left them, all power to exert themselves to leave departed. The only door that seemed open for escape was that of suicide. The men who kept these women, as well as the gamblers and saloon men, were always ready to pay a high fee for professional services.

Another large phase of my practice was that of bringing new citizens into Spindle-Top oil field. One night a workman came for me in a hurry. He told me that he needed me in his home and needed me at once. We left immediately and soon came to what was called a tent-shack. The floor of planks was laid flat on the ground. The simple room, twelve feet square, was boarded up four feet high with rough, twelve-inch planks and covered with a tarpaulin. One opening in front served for both windows and doorway. This room was used for living, dining, sleeping and cooking for the family. At the moment I arrived, which was just two minutes ahead of the stork, it was being used as the delivery room. A woman in the first stages of labor lay on a sagging cot. Underneath her was a dirty, torn sheet, and over her an old, filthy quilt.

A little oil lamp, without a chimney, sent out a flickering, feeble light. There was neither hot water nor towels, and no semblance of cleanliness or sanitation. A smoking fire of wet wood smouldered in the rusted, broken stove. An old woman, ignorant and unwashed, was present, but she might as well have been absent so far as any assistance she was to me. I had not been used to delivering women under such conditions, but the mother was a strong, young, backwoods woman and the baby came all right.

Following that night I had many similar calls, and under practically the same conditions. Sometimes the woman did not even have a shack to live in; many times it was a tent with a dirt floor in which she brought her young into the world. So many of the men drank and gambled that their wives and babies were often without enough to eat and wear, to say nothing of having anything ready or sanitary for the new-born life.

I tried to instruct the women in sanitation, the care of themselves, the danger of mosquitoes and flies. Malaria took a large toll of my patients. But the rush of riches into eager hands, the lawlessness, lust, and the intoxication of the wild excitement caused most of my advice and teaching to fall on careless and deaf ears.

A few months after I had located in Spindle-Top, one night a rap came on the door of my room at the hotel as I was lying on my bed for a few minutes' rest. I groaned in my spirit when I heard that rap, for I knew it meant a call. I opened the door, and there stood a half-drunk, dirty-looking man, rain dripping from his hat and the tatters of his coat.

He said that he wanted me to go at once to the oil field and take care of his wife. He explained that he had no money then but would pay me as soon as he could. I got my bag and we started. The rain was coming down in torrents. You could feel the darkness, it was so black. We stumbled and floundered through the mud, stepping into holes filled with water, sliding and slipping, before we finally came to his tent.

When he pulled back the flap of his tent and we entered, I gasped. In one corner was an old broken cook stove, standing on pieces of brick, its rusty stove pipe almost falling apart. Not a spark of fire was in it. In the center of the room stood a home-made table covered with dirty dishes, and a dish pan full of dark, greasy water, with the limp, filthy dish-rag hanging over its side. Two broken chairs and a rickety packing box, on which stood an oil lamp with a smoky chimney obscuring the light it might have given, completed the furnishings.

Over in another corner, on an old, unpainted iron bed, lay a large woman. A mop of uncombed, drab, yellow hair hung around a face tougher looking than some of the faces of the women I had seen plying their trade in the gambling houses.

This was to be her first baby. She was in labor and had been alone in the tent while her husband had gone for me. I beat the stork by just one jump. The look she gave us from those little green eyes of hers, and the choice curses with which she greeted her husband, made me realize that at least I had an interesting patient, if not a gentle or cultured one. When I had made a preliminary examination I saw the urgency of the situation and asked her husband whether he had any hot water or clean towels. There was neither. The sheets and old quilt on the bed evidently had never been washed. Her pains were growing more frequent and harder, and her curses louder. She cursed her husband for getting her into her present condition and cursed me for not getting her out of it.

By this time I was realizing in full the fact that I had been called to a labor case. Her husband stood in the middle of the tent. His old wet hat was pushed back on his head; his hands were in his frayed pockets; a cigarette hung from his half-open mouth. He did not have enough sober sense left to make a fire in the stove. One can imagine the joyful anticipation I had when, after another examination, I found a knee presentation instead of a normal delivery.

That woman and I worked for hours trying to have that baby. The husband finally sat down in the broken chair, tilted it back against the old box, and went to sleep, uninterested in the curses the woman poured out on him, her unborn baby, and her doctor. The uneasy feeling which had assailed me earlier in the evening when I entered the tent increased with the prospects for delivery. Someone was going to have the job of bathing and dressing a new citizen of Spindle-Top, and I was not a candidate for the office.

I awakened the new papa, for I was trying to figure out which one of us was going to wash and dress the baby. When the cursing and groaning woman was delivered, I picked up the baby, shoved her into the father's hands before he could protest, and said,"Here, take your baby." Once he had her in his hands, I felt easier, for I was almost sure I would not have to take her back and wash and dress her. His face was a study in emotions, for the baby was not a very pleasant looking object. He looked down at her and began a stream of oaths.

As I saw that the mother had relaxed and drifted off to sleep, I picked up my bag and hat and started to leave. When the panic-stricken father recognized my intentions, he yelled, "Hey! Yuh... Yuh... Yuh... ca... ca.... can't go. What are you going to do with it?" I replied that I was not going to do anything with it, as there was neither oil nor grease in the tent, it would be his privilege and pleasure to wash and dress his baby. I edged toward the flap of the tent, and he began to whine, beg, and swear.

Finally, when he realized that he made no impression on me, he said, "Wait, Doc, don't go. I gotta proposition to make yuh. I'll shoot yuh the best two out of three and give yuh a horse and, the guy what loses, dresses the kid." I was thinking fast. I was afraid that he would arouse his wife and I did not know what would be the result if she decided to sit in with us on the conference about who should wash the baby. I thought that with one to go and his drunken and excited state, I could beat him and save further argument. I agreed, but I did not retrace my steps. He laid the baby quietly down on the bed, tiptoed over to where I was waiting for him and rubbed his hands on his trousers.

Fishing into his pocket, he brought out two well-worn dice, and we got down on our knees in the dirt, where the floor should have been. Caressing the dice in his hands, he talked and begged them to win for him in the most pleading and pitiful voice I had ever heard. With a soft groan he shot first; but his pleading was in vain, for they rolled him "low."

I took the dice, shook them, and threw "high." I looked up at him just in time to see a fixed look of horror come into his face as his mouth fell open. I turned to see what he was staring at and met his wife's eyes. She was looking in wild-eyed fury at both of us then she burst out into a volley of the most torrid curses I had ever heard. The names she called us were beyond my comprehension as she told us where to go and what to do when we got there. I reached for my hat and bag and said to him, "I won." And as I went out under the flap of the tent, my sense of humor returned, and I whispered, "GOOD NIGHT."

Spindle-Top Burns

One night, about one o'clock in the morning, I awoke with a start from a deep sleep. Outside my window there was a great commotion. My room was filled with light. People were running in the streets, cursing, yelling, and crying. Alarmed, I reached for my clothes and somehow got them on. The crack of pistol shots rent the air. Just as I finished dressing, there was an explosion which rocked the earth. My heart almost stood still from fright, as I ran out on the street. It seemed that Judgment Day had come, and the world must be burning up.

I asked a white-faced, wild-eyed man running past me what had happened. He replied that a steel oil tank had blown up and the Spindle-Top field was on fire. Bang! Crash! Boom! Explosion after explosion followed, as large and small tanks and derricks went up like dynamite. The sky was a sea of flame. Tongues of fire shot hundreds of feet into the air.

The dense, rolling smoke curled itself into fantastic shapes. Great quantities of gas formed livid balls of fire which exploded and burst into flames high in the air. Flames, twisting and writhing like hell-tossed snakes, leaped from derricks, pump-houses, and shacks, leaving them flaming torches as they passed.

Hard-faced men sobbed and wept like babies as they watched their wealth vanish in an instant. Women screaming, crying and dragging children or some piece of valued furniture, rushed to safety. Orders and countermand orders were hurled through the air. Men, wild with fear, tried to save their tanks, wells, derricks, homes, and places of business only to be relentlessly pushed back by the mocking flames. That night was never to be forgotten. The news of the fire spread. Within a few hours people began to pour into the field from Beaumont and other places. Some of them were owners of leases, well-rigs, and stores, many of which were already destroyed. All that stood in the pathway of the fire was doomed. Nothing could stop the roaring flames as they licked hungrily at everything perishable.

People sought frantically for their families and friends. On the ground lay the burned, injured, and dead. Men and women were trying to relieve the suffering ones, or were carrying them to places where they might be cared for. My office was crowded with the injured, burned, hysterical men and women, their nerves broken with the loss of their fortunes. I worked feverishly over my patients and was soon staggering with fatigue. As soon as I had the burned flesh, broken bones, or torn limbs treated and sedatives administered where they were needed, the groans and cries of those still unattended caused me to continue to aid them mechanically though my tired mind had almost ceased to function. Toward morning I had the office cleared and, locking the door, I fell on my operating table and was soon in a drug-like sleep.

A loud pounding on the door finally pulled me back from the oblivion of stupor. I groped my way to the door and blinked in the bright sunlight. There stood a crowd of prescriptions, they told me that they were going to Sour Lake or Saratoga. Within a few days Spindle-Top was practically deserted and my practice was almost completely gone. The exodus from Spindle-Top was both rapid and complete. Life had become so exciting for me both as to experience and earning money, that the increasing quiet of the place made me nervous. I decided to join the hegira. I did not know where to reach the old doctor who, evidently, was still on his drunk. One day I turned the office over to the druggist and went to Beaumont. There I bought a supply of medicines and instruments and an operating table. Without a backward glance at burned-out Spindle-Top, I gaily left for Sour Lake and Saratoga.

I looked over both fields, for two or three days and, deciding that I liked Saratoga better, I located there. A gusher had been brought in, a real wildcat, in wildcat territory.

Saratoga looked like a wildcat to me in more ways than in oil wells. It was an old town located in that part of Texas known as the "Big Thicket." To reach it, one went to Kuntz and there took a hack twelve miles over the roughest road imaginable. I thought that the road from Beaumont to Spindle-Top had been rough, but I found that it was a paved highway compared to the road to Saratoga. It was literally made up of mud-holes, ruts, sand, and roots of trees. As far as I could see, the town consisted of an old, two-story, frame building which looked as if it had been made in the year 1901 or 1902. Two large rooms downstairs, with a wide hall dividing them, two large rooms upstairs, a rambling gallery running the whole length of the house both front and back, completed the dilapidated place. About ten yards behind this place stood an equally shabby, old, one-story house, which was used for the dining room and kitchen. The dining room was connected with the main part of the house by a narrow board walk.

Immense pine trees surrounded the house, making a picturesque setting for it. This unsightly place had the pretentious name of "The Hotel Saratoga." Two other houses, an old log and an old general store, which supplied the few families living in the "Big Thicket" and those living at Batson Prairie, six miles away, completed Saratoga.

I look over this metropolis for a place for a drugstore and office. I found that an enterprising native had built a long room on one side of the general store. He was using the front part of this room for a cold drink stand and the back of it for a store-room. I persuaded him to rent me the back room, for it was the only one I could get in the town. Placing my drugs in it, I hung out my sign of M. D., and was ready for business.

The big companies had already established quite a camp in the "Thicket." Crews of men worked feverishly to clear away the jungle, build derricks, tank-farms, and pump stations.

It was only a few days after I opened up that a mad rush of people poured into the town and began buying leases as wildly as they had at Spindle-Top. Like a mushroom the boom town sprang up, and we were off again for more wild, hectic days I realized that my judgment had been correct. I was in on the ground floor, the first doctor in Saratoga with the only drug-store in the new oil field.

A saw-mill was soon set up and running. It operated day and night, cutting derrick timbers and lumber for the new buildings of Saratoga. Mule and ox-teams began coming with heavy machinery, pipe, and all kinds of oil-field supplies.

Daily, men arrived with supplies of whiskey and beer. In the absence of gambling-houses, tents were set up and in them the saloons and gambling places started business. Tarpaulins spread on the ground took the place of gambling tables.

A little saw-mill could not supply lumber fast enough. Another one was brought in. Soon it also was working to its full capacity. Often it was but a few hours from the time the stately tree growing in the forest became a plank in the walls of a gambling house, "Tommy-joint," or a saloon.

By the time the first rush was started, the girls and their pimps began arriving, and more and more came until there was a small town of them. Although the little saw-mills were working as fast as they could, many people had to live in tents for months, and even the saloons and prostitutes carried on their business in tents. As quickly as men could hammer the planks in place, saloons, stores, residences, gambling houses, and red-light shacks sprang up.

Suddenly awake, the old hotel took on a new lease of life with a new coat of paint, thereby entering into the spirit of the moment. Those of us who had no families had a place to go, eat, sleep and call home. Of course, such conveniences as baths, toilets, running water and telephone were lacking, but we got along very well.

In the cook-shack, behind the hotel, the "chefs" dished up so much Irish stew that I got so I could hardly look an Irishman in the face. The merchants, saloon-men, gambling house owners, drillers, rough-necks, contractors, lease owners and the doctor ate at a long table in a shed at the side of the cook-shack with its dirt floor and benches without backs. In other parts of the field each company had its own cook-shack whose "chefs" dished up Irish stew to the workmen.

By far the most interesting eating place in the field was a long shed on the other side of the creek where a large colored woman fed the gamblers, whores and pimps of the town. She was about five feet tall, five and a half feet around, and blacker than night, except for the glistening white of her eyes and teeth. She had a voice like a siren with a range comparable to that of a fog horn. When she threw her kinky head back, opened her mouth, and yelled, "Come and git it," it always seemed to me that she was talking to no one group of persons in particular, but to the whole town in general.

One day the old darky got sick and sent for me. Long before I reached the tent, I could hear her praying. When I entered, she was lying with her face to the side of the tent. I spoke to her and she turned her head about halfway around, opened her eyes, which looked like two large snowballs with a dark spot on each of them, and said, "Lawdy, Lawdy, Doctah, git me well and outa heah. Ah doan wants ter die and let de Lawd find out Ah's bin cookin fer all dese bad wimmins. Fo den sho nuf nevah would He let dis pore ol nigga eben look at dem golen streets."

In a few days I had the old Negro up and, true to humanity, white or black, she forgot all about her fear of not reaching Heaven and went right back to cooking for "dem bad wimmins."

She had been in the kitchen a few days when she again sent for me. When I went into the place, she took me into her own private little tent by the side of her kitchen, and there in the center of it stood a small table. It was set with a clean, white cloth, and on it was a great platter of golden brown fried chicken with all the trimmings, such as I had not seen for many a day. It was her token of appreciation to the doctor for keeping her a time longer from missing "dem golen streets."

Camps and derricks were being built over such a wide area that getting to them, especially on emergency calls, of which so much of my practice consisted, became a serious problem for me. Events happened quickly in the oil field. Gushers blew in, towns were built over night and abandoned as quickly, and accidents and death kept pace with the insane occurrences of those days.

My work carried me far and near over the field. When it was a case of life and death, it meant my sparing neither myself nor my animal. I soon had the reputation of answering a call in record time. A livery stable was opened and I thought my problem was solved, for now I could rent a horse when I needed one. It worked all right for a time but, finally, the livery man complained that I was running his horses to death and he would not rent one to me. I did not know what to do, but at this time Fortune favored me. A man drove into Saratoga overland. His outfit included a horse of race stock for which he had no particular use because of its hellish disposition. When I learned that he had this horse for sale, I purchased it. It proved to be just what I was looking for as it had speed and endurance to carry me on my rounds.

One afternoon I was called on a labor case. The woman lived in a tent. A short distance away in another tent a man, about sixty years of age, was gambling with some others. The woman was in the third stages of labor when an argument arose over the honesty of the gamblers and a fight followed. In the heat of battle one of the gamblers drew a long, sharp, knife, reached over, and with a quick slash, let the old man's bowels out through the walls of his belly. I heard the cursing and the thuds of the blows struck and the scream of the wounded man but, being used to such things, I had paid no attention to them.

Just as the child was being presented, I heard a commotion at the door of the tent. The women who were standing guard was telling someone in emphatic voices that he could not enter. My attention being at last arrested, I looked around just in time to see a man staggering into the tent holding the lower part of his belly, a quantity of blood pouring out over his arm.

"Doc!" he cried. "My guts are cut out. Do something for me quick!"

I called to the gamblers who were with him to take him to my office, that I would be there immediately. In a few minutes the child was born and, turning the rest of the affair over to the old ladies, I grabbed my bag and rushed across to the office. The patient was laid out on the operating table, blood everywhere and his bowels lying outside of his body. I soon got his intestines untangled and pushed back inside him where they belonged and sewed him up. I told his gambler friends to bring the homemade stretcher. We moved him to it from the operating table and I told them to carry him with as much care as possible to the tent where he lived, lay him on his bed and not let him move until I saw him again.

What prevented that knife from cutting through the intestines, I have never been able to explain.

SARATOGA

Saratoga was soon a booming oil town with the customary excitement of work, gambling, fighting, drunkenness, pimping, and whoring that go with such places.

One night, just as I was about to retire, there was a knock at my door. I opened it and there stood a tall, dark complexioned man with shifty, crocodile eyes, and a devil in each of them. The well-cut, blue suit and white shirt were not the dress of the oil man, merchant, gambler, pimp, roughneck or anyone else in the oil field. His pistol-belt and scabbard were made of a better grade leather than the usual run of belts.

I had been in the oil field long enough by this time to get bravely over being surprised at anything. I told the man to come in and asked him what I could do for him.

In the voice of a gentleman he said, "Doctor, I have never had the pleasure of meeting you, but I have watched you in action at Spindle-Top and here, and I have wanted to meet you. I think we are going to be friends. Just call me Mac. I am a sporting man from Beaumont." He looked me squarely in the eyes. I had heard of this man, "Mac." As he stood before me, his fantastic reputation ran through my mind. He was one of the two men in that part of the country who had a reputation of never having failed to knock a man down when he hit him with his pistol.

"You are out of your class with this bunch of sons-of-bitches, and so am I," he continued. "I am a university graduate and my people do not know that I am here in this kind of business. I came to Beaumont with the oil boom. The excitement and money got me. I am playing it heavily, and I am going to put in one of the finest gambling houses in this part of the country and operate all through the oil fields."

I told him that I was a doctor, and a doctor was not out of place anywhere that he was alleviating pain.

"Well, I don't believe you were ever used to the type of practice you have here, and it is going to get rougher than anything you have ever seen or heard about."

It was not difficult to tell by his speech that he was highly educated and of good breeding. But easy money and a streak of wild blood had been the cause of his entering the profession of gambling. He built a large saloon, gambling house and a whorehouse in one-half block of my office.

On his opening night he invited the public to be his guests and drink all the whiskey they wanted "on the house." By ten o'clock the place was crowded to overflowing so that one could hardly elbow his way through. The new gramophone he had brought from Beaumont ground out its music.

Rough-necks, drillers, lease-owners, oil contractors, business men, whores, and pimps thronged the place. By twelve o'clock the whiskey was getting in its effects. Girls, partially drunk, slipped money from the pockets of drunken men as they leaned against them affectionately. Fights were started over the women. Arguments over a fancied wrong, or often over nothing but whiskey, inflamed passion. In the gambling room men gambled away oil wells, leases worth a fortune and thousands of dollars in money. As the owner was his own floor-walker, he would not permit the noisy "drunks" of the saloon to enter the gambling department. He knew that if they got back there concentration on the games would cease, and it was there that he was making his money. Before opening his house, Mac had sent me word that he wished me to care for anyone injured in his place and he would pay the bill.

That night, when the drunks got too rough, he tried to get them to go home. If they insisted on staying and refused to behave, he would take out his old black forty-five pistol and tap the offenders on the head. Then he would call his bouncers and have those he had knocked out carried to my place for repairs.

I did not get to bed the night of his opening. My office was crowded with people from his saloon in different states of

injury; some cut up with knives, others needing broken nos-
es repaired, or rapidly swelling black eyes treated. Many of
them had to have a few stitches taken in their scalps where
Mac's gun had cut through when he hit them. But his opening night was a success financially for him and for me.

The famous Teel Acre was drilled. A man had leased one
acre of it from the family, put a well down in one corner
of the acre, and it came in, a gusher. Then he located three
other wells, one in each of the other corners, with the same
results. People went mad. Other drillers crowded the line of
this acre, and a forest of derricks sprang up. They were over
a pool of oil. In their wild haste to get a gusher some of them
lost their wells, but the majority became millionaires.

Oil wells and gushers came in one after another. Drilling,
gushers shooting their liquid gold into the air, gas blowouts
causing derricks and tools to be lost, all made a wild picture.
Fearful that other oil men might crowd their lines, the owners of the leases, or one of their employees stood guard over
their land with shot guns in their hands, as they worked
in mad haste to get their wells down first and get the oil as
fast as possible. They knew that with the derricks so close
to each other, it was only a question of time until someone's
well would be a dry hole.

When the town of Saratoga was being built, citizens forgot
to erect a jail. As the oil excitement spread and more gamblers, saloon keepers, whores, gun-men, and crooks came
in, crime increased. The deputy sheriff kept things in hand
fairly well, but it was a problem to know what to do with his
prisoners. Many of the arrests were for drinking or fighting.
In despair, the sheriff finally decided to establish a jail for
his prisoners. One night he sent for me to come and treat
one of the prisoners he had locked up. He told me to come
to the general store and he would take me to the prisoner.
I went over and met the deputy sheriff. On one side of the
store was a small clearing with a few small pine trees left
here and there. The sheriff had sent for a lot of hand cuffs.
There, handcuffed to one of those trees, was the maddest

man I had ever seen. In a drunken fight he had been beaten rather severely. He was bleeding from a scalp wound and a cut on the face.

The sheriff had solved his jail problem by leading his prisoners up to one of those trees in the little clearing and handcuffing their hands around it. They would curse, cry and beg, but as the whiskey died out and sleep overtook them, they would slip down to the ground and go to sleep their heads on one side, their legs doubled up, their arms embraced around the tree. The sentences given the prisoners depended on the extent of their guilt. I felt that the sheriff had proved that "Necessity is the mother of invention."

Tough Guys

At about seven o'clock one morning there came a knock on my door. I called out, "Who is it?"

A rough voice answered, "Open up, Doc."

I opened the door and there stood the owner of one of the toughest joints in the oil field, a thick, short heavy man with shaggy hair and stubby, black moustache, who was called "Two Gun Bill." With him was another man whom I knew as "Long Jim," a tall, rangy, rawboned man whose hair fell over his beady eyes. They were both talking at the same time, telling me to hurry up and come with them at once.

I said, "Pipe down and tell me what is the matter."

I knew from the state of excitement they were in that it must be something serious, for these two birds were tough. Then they told me that there had been a fight at the joint and Jim Bezel had the whole top of his head lying wide open, and the blood spurting like a gusher. At the name of Jim Bezel I felt sick at the stomach, for I had watched him in action in the saloons, gambling joints, and whorehouses, and he was one of the men I had met that I always hoped I would never have to work on. However I grabbed my emergency surgical bag, and away we went. When we arrived at the joint, a ring of the toughest looking characters I had ever seen outside the "Pen" was around the killer. He and the man who had hit him had an argument. The gun-man was drunk. As the argument increased, the killer made a move for his gun, but he was not quick enough on the draw. The other chap jerked out his old forty-five, took it in both hands and, rising up on his tip-toes, cracked down on Jim Bezel's head with all his strength. The killer went down and out like a light. While he lay unconscious, the other fellow made fast time getting away from there.

The blood which had poured from one side of the unconscious man's head made it look as if there had been a hog killing. The table, benches, the dirt floor, and his clothes were soaked with it. He had been unconscious for such a

long time that the toughs in the gambling-joint thought
he was not coming to. By the time I arrived, he was re-
vived and was half-sitting up, in his hand a gun which
looked as long as my leg. Little shifty, light-blue eyes,
blood-shot and with an expression of fear and murder
peered out at me from under light eyelashes and a big
gash in his skull. A crooked, narrow, cruel mouth was
emitting a stream of oaths and threats. Waving his gun in
the air, he emphasized the fact that he was going to kill
the "damned son-of-a-bitch" as soon as I stopped this
"damned bleeding."

His mean, hard-looking face was white with fear that
he was going to die. Like most killers, he was yellow
when he faced death. He was certain that he was going to
bleed to death and I encouraged him in this belief as best
I could. Telling him to sit down on a bench beside one of
the gambling tables, I got one of the men to bring me a
pan of hot water. As I opened my bag, I told him to put
his pistol down, but he said that he would be damned if
he would, for if that son-of-a-bitch came in he was going
to kill him.

I did not know what to do, for I knew I must stop the
hemorrhage, and soon, if he was going to live. I started
to operate on him with that gun still in his drunken, murderous hand. He continued to keep up a steady stream
of threats against the men's lives whom he had fought
with, and especially the one who had hit him, punctuating each of his curses with a wave of his gun. When the
gun-waving and cursing renewed the blood spurting, he
turned white with fear and began to whine and beg me
not to let him die. This went on for awhile until I saw that
I was getting nowhere with the operation.

Beginning to see red with rage myself, I laid my instruments down and said, "You big, yellow, drunken son-of-
a-bitch, put that gun down and put it down *now*."

A gasp went up from the on-lookers, because no one
had ever before talked to him like that. Half-mad, half-

scared, he cursed me and said that he wasn't going to do it.

"All right, you drunken, murdering bastard," I answered, "I am going to let you bleed to death." And I started to pick up my instruments.

When he thought I was going, he began to whine and cry and promised to put the gun down. To show me that he meant business, he laid it down between his feet. I was standing behind him. The ground on which I stood sloped a bit, so I was a little higher than he. I started to cut his hair away from the wound. While I worked, I noticed his head slowly leaning forward. Thinking that he had fallen asleep, I worked with all speed to get him sewed up before he awoke. Looking down to see whether or not he was sound asleep, I saw him, at that instant, bending lower, with his hand closing over his pistol. I stopped, put my instruments down, and reached over and took his pistol away from him.

Calling the proprietor of the gambling-joint, I gave him the pistol and told him to keep it until I had finished sewing up the patient. My actions so frightened those thugs who were standing watching me that they almost left the place. I was so mad that I had forgotten all about his being a killer. I reached round and took his chin in my right hand, twisted his head with a rough jerk and clamped my arm on his head so that he could not move, turning his head until the wound was directly in front of me. Since I operate with my left hand, I was now able to work. He was trying to curse me, but I clamped a little tighter and shut off that cursing almost altogether.

All who had not left by this time had stopped their gambling and drinking and were watching to see what would happen. When they saw that the killer did not have his gun and what a nice hold I had on him, they watched and kidded him a few minutes; then they all went back to their interrupted gambling and drinking.

I had my needles all threaded before I took his gun away from him, so I started my one-handed operation. By this time I was mad and thoroughly enjoying the operation. I picked up a needle, shoved it into his scalp until I felt the point ram into his skull. He jumped, howled, and cursed. I pulled it back out of the skull, set it under the other side of the cut exactly where I wanted it to come through, and repeated the procedure. And I was not very gentle with him. The scalp was so tough and elastic that when I shoved my needle up, it would stretch, but eventually the needle would force its way through so that I could tie the stitches.

As I pulled the first stitch together, he let out such a blood-curdling yell and oath one might have thought that he was being killed. The gamblers, thugs, pimps, and drillers decided that he was dying, with joy left their gambling, and came running with all speed to see it happen.

I took several stitches in the wound, setting the needle through the scalp in the same manner as the first time. Before I got through, he was cursing the human race in general and me in particular. He told me that I was the first one he was going to kill as soon as I had finished the operation and he had been turned loose with his pistol. I paid him no attention and never released his head until I got the stitches all set. I knew that I could tie those stitches and dress the wound before he could move his head, for it had been in that cramped position so long. After I turned him loose it would take him quite some time to get his neck limbered up enough to go into action. Working as fast as I could I had the stitches all tied and the wound dressed before he started calling for his pistol.

While I was cleaning up my instruments, he took his pistol, threw the cylinder out to see that it was loaded, cocked it, and let the hammer down several times.

One of the gamblers who had lain down on a bench near where I was operating had fallen into a drunken sleep. The killer had the body of the pistol in his hand and was pulling the hammer back and letting it down. Suddenly the gambler, who was lying on his back, awoke. The killer was standing immediately in front of him. The gambler looked up and right into the barrel of the pistol just as the killer cocked it., He made one flop, off the bench he went, hit the ground, rolled over and over, under the side of the tent and into the night.

After Bezel had satisfied himself that his little "pet" was in perfect working order, he turned to me and said, "I am going back to town with you."

I made no objection to this unalluring suggestion, for the self-invited guest was again waving his old black pistol in the air. I picked up my instrument case, and we started out of the tent.

Just as we got outside he said, "Wait, Doc, I forgot my hat," and stepped back.

When he disappeared into the tent, I decided that I did not want the pleasure of his company back to town. I stepped out into the dark so that when he returned he could not see me.

He began calling and cursing, which did not give me much inclination to answer him, and the louder he called, "Doctor, you son-of-a-bitch, come back here," the less I desired his company.

By that time I was far enough away that I knew he was not going back to town with me, and I hoped that he would be dead or sober the next time I saw him. In either condition he would be less dangerous and easier to deal with than at that time.

I Am Introduced To Batson Prairie

One day a man came into my office and asked me to go with him to see a patient at Batson Prairie. I had never been to Batson, but I had heard such wild stories about the place, the road over there and the people, I was not enthusiastic at the thought of the trip. However I told him that I would go. He said that he would wait for me until I could clear my office of patients. I got as much of the history of the patient as I could from him and packed my bag with what I thought I would need. As there was not another drug store within a radius of twenty-five miles, it was necessary for me to carry my drugs and surgical equipment with me.

There was a semblance of a road that the oil companies had cut through the thicket in order to carry oil machinery, pipe, and supplies into their camps. We left this so-called road and were soon riding through the jungle-like Big Thicket. The trees were crowded so close that we could ride only single-file through them on a narrow trail. Rain was falling, and the ground was soggy and swampy. We crossed several small streams where our horses sank down nearly to their bellies in muddy water. Then we came to the Bayou, a slow, sluggish body of water, the largest stream between Saratoga and Batson Prairie. My friend called to me to keep my horse well to the right or he might bog down. He then started across the Bayou, my horse following his. Suddenly my horse started to rear and plunge and thoughts of a muddy grave passed through my mind, but I finally got him quiet, and we crossed over.

Just as we got across the stream, I heard a strange and terrifying noise. My companion called to me to hurry up, stuck spurs to his horse and was off in a dead run. My horse seemed to sense that something exciting was taking place, and he started to gallop. I leaned over on my saddle to avoid being dragged off by the low-hanging limbs of the trees, the vines and briers catching and tearing at my hands, face, and clothing, while I tried with all my strength to stop my horse.

On we dashed, and soon I had overtaken my companion, who had stopped and taken out his pistol. He told me to listen. It seemed that the Big Thicket was on the move and going to run over us.

We sat on our horses and waited. Suddenly, big, little and middle-sized hogs burst out of the thicket and crossed our trail, running as if their lives depended on their speed. Some seventy-five or a hundred crossed the trail, squealing and grunting. They passed like a roaring wave. One small hog could not keep up with the others; as it started across the trail, a large, dark, moving shape, directly behind it, jumped on it, raised its front paw like a huge hammer, and brought it down on its head. The pig squealed with fear and pain and sank down on the ground. My companion raised his pistol and began firing at the black shape but, at the noise of the pistol, it bounded away into the thicket and disappeared. My horse was plunging and rearing so that I could hardly see what was happening but, as the animal ran past me, I saw that it was a bear.

As we rode on, my companion told me that the hogs belonged to the people living in the big thicket. The owners did not corral them or feed them, as was customary, but let them roam the thicket, foraging for themselves. When winter came, the owners would locate a place, build great pens out of small logs and, for a month or two, keep corn scattered around and in these places. The hogs would come for miles to get the corn. When all the hogs had collected near the pens, a day would be set and all the men and boys would gather with their long-eared hounds, surround the hogs, and start the drive. The hogs were wild and, as the men, boys, and dogs closed in on them, they would break for the thicket.

The dogs baying and barking, the men and boys on their galloping horses, shooting their pistols and yelling, would try to drive the running animals into the pens. At the openings of these were long arms built of logs extending out on each side. When the hogs came to one of these arms, they would run along it and go into the pen. Those that went into the pens the owners would divide equally among themselves. The wilder ones the dogs would catch by the ears and hold until someone had killed them or tied them to take them back to the pen. Often a boar would break the dog's hold on his ear, at the same time slashing at him with his murderous tusks. If the hog struck him, the dog might be scattered all over the thicket. If the dog escaped death, he never again made the mistake of attacking a wild boar.

We finally reached a little open space about the size of a garden, and my companion informed me that this was the beginning of Batson Prairie. We rode a little farther and came to another clearing in which was a plank house, built upon stilts with cracks between the planks wide enough to admit air and light. In that hot, sultry thicket, air was thought more necessary than chinking up the openings. The mosquitoes were so large that they had to enter via the door.

As we approached the house a pack of hounds, their ears almost reaching the ground, came yelping to meet us. As they came running toward us, my companion told me about the virtues of each. They were so strong that they could hold a hog five times their weight. I looked at their ribs showing through the skin, and I thought that each should go to the big thicket, catch a hog five times its weight and eat it every bit. When my companion saw me looking at their ribs, he explained that if they were fat, they could not hold out to run the hogs down.

We went up four or five sagging, broken steps, crossed a wide gallery, and entered an immense living room, with floors and walls of rough, unpainted planks. In one end of the room was a great fireplace beneath a crude, heavy piece of timber which served as a mantel. On this stood a beautiful antique clock, no doubt an heirloom brought over by the forefathers of these settlers. A large home-made table in the middle of the room and a few home-made chairs constituted the furniture. An old lady with finely chiseled features, showing the good blood of her ancestors, greeted us. She was clothed in coarse, home-made clothes and wore heavy, thick shoes. From the thin, well-molded lips there hung a stick tooth brush from which dripped a thin, brown stream of saliva and snuff. She asked me in a high-pitched, nasal voice if I was the new doctor from the city. I answered, "Guilty," and she smilingly led me into a small bedroom.

On a crude, home-made bed lay an old man with a heavy brush of grey hair and tobacco-stained whiskers, which came down to his chest. From his looks I thought that he might be the "grand-daddy" of Batson Prairie—men, hogs, dogs, bear, and all. I found him suffering from a gunshot wound which he had received several weeks past in an argument with pistols. He had met his opponent of an old feud of generations standing. When I touched the question of how it happened, the steely, suspicious look in the old grey eyes informed me that I was a "furriner," and on ground I had no right to tread. He refused to take any anaesthetic and stood the painful operation without complaint or wincing. I left instructions and medicine with him and told him that I would return the third day. The rugged constitution, simple living, and clean thinking told in the old man's case. In two weeks he was up and about and ready to finish the argument at anytime that he crossed the pathway of the man who had shot him.

More Gushers

One night, not long after my trip to Batson Prairie, two of the best known drillers from Spindle-Top came into my drug store for medicine. They told me that they were on their way to Batson Prairie to drill a "wild-cat." I told them that I had been to Batson Prairie and, in my opinion, any "cat" they ran into over there would be a "wild" one.

A few weeks later a son of the old man who had "shot it out" in a long-standing feud and had been wounded, came into my office. In the course of conversation he told me that his father was all right, and that two drillers had put down a wildcat on his father's land. It had come in a gusher, and I was invited to come over and see it.

Two days later three friends of mine came by the office and said, "Doc, we're all going over to Batson Prairie to see that gusher. Don't you want to give the undertaker a chance to make some money? If you do, come on and go with us."

I protested that I could not go because there were too many calls in rapid succession from accidents in the field, and too many sick people needing my care. But all my objections were talked down, and I was delighted to find my friends could think of so many convincing arguments to still my annoying conscience. I closed my office, left a sign on the door, "Urgent call. Will be back later" and, mounting my horse, I rode off to Batson Prairie.

When we arrived at the well, the gusher was shut down, and all the crew was gone; so that there was nothing to see but the derrick and the crew's tent where the men ate and slept. As we approached the derrick of this gusher, a man stepped out with a double-barreled shot gun across his arm and ordered us to stop. One of the men in our party recognized the guard and called out, "Hello Bill! What are you doing here?"

The guard then invited us to approach. We found ourselves standing on the floor of the derrick of the first oil well in Batson Prairie, a field destined to have the most poisonous gas of all fields in the South Texas district. I stayed and talked a few hours with the people in Batson and returned to my practice.

The following Sunday I returned to Batson to see a patient. Out on the edge of a small clearing near this same derrick a town was springing up. From Saratoga, Houston, Sour Lake, and other places had already flocked over a thousand adventurers. Since Wednesday of the week before when I had been there several more derricks had been started. On each side of a so-called street stood a row of tents in which men were selling whiskey, playing cards, rolling dice and gambling their money away on the tarpaulins, which had been spread on the dirt floor. But all seemed as contented and happy as if they were seated on comfortable chairs at hardwood tables.

About a hundred yards from these tents were three or four other tents clustered together. This group constituted what was known as "Ann's Place," and belonged to a famous prostitute who operated one of the largest houses of ill repute in the oil fields. She had not had time to get beds for her girls, but they did not let such little inconveniences deprive them of their business.

The following Sunday morning I was called again to see a patient in Batson Prairie. As I rode into town it seemed that pandemonium reigned. In the clearing, slightly larger than a baseball diamond, which my companion, son of the old man, had told me a few weeks before was Batson Prairie, there now stood a motley array of shacks, coaches, buggies, and spring wagons, drawn by mules and horses of every description. To one little half spring-wagon, half buggy, were hitched an ox and a poor little pony. Business men, drillers, drunks, pimps and their women, gamblers, gunmen, and girls from Ann's Place elbowed their way through the crowds cursing and swearing, their ribald laughter and obscene greetings scorching the air. The blazing sun and flying dust added to the discomfort of the crowd.

Two or three saloons and a few restaurants, devoid of any semblance of wall or roof, stood under the great trees. Flies were feasting on the food and the drinks which the people stood consuming, but everyone seemed to be doing a rushing business. The sound of gamblers' voices begging the dice to win for them, the hum of men's and women's voices bargaining for leases or arranging for wells to be drilled, the coarse soliciting and shrill laughter of the prostitutes, the curses, thuds of blows, as men settled or unsettled their disputes, ripped to shreds the peace of the Sunday morning. Not a hotel, house, or shack was there to offer a bed to those thousands of people. The only hopes of places for them to sleep were the wagons, hacks, tents, or ground.

The patient I had been called to see was an oil lease man. He had a big tent for an office. On one side of it he had hung a large blueprint from which he was selling oil leases as fast as he could take in the earnest money and write the receipts.

When I appeared he said to me in a whisper, "Doctor, come in. I have a bad throat. I must have my voice for the next few days. I shall need it as I have never before needed it in my life."

I examined his throat and told him that I could do very little for him unless he stopped talking and permitted it to rest.

He looked at me with beseeching eyes and said, "But Doctor, I have to talk and you must help me."

I told him that I could prepare some medicine to shrink the swollen mucous membrane of the throat so that he could talk a bit, but that was the best I could do. He pleaded with me to hurry with my treatment so that he could get back to the selling of his oil leases. I swabbed his throat and told him not to speak for a few minutes.

He waited for about two minutes, swallowed, and said, in a pleased but hoarse voice, "Doctor, I can talk! You stay here and wait. When my voice quits on me again, I will be back. You keep swabbing my throat and keep me talking until this rush is over."

I sat down on a box, and he again started selling his leases. About every fifteen minutes his voice would fail, and I again would swab his throat. I stayed two days with him and he paid me well for my time, but I watched him make more money those two days than I could hope to make in my profession in years.

In Saratoga, also, more wells were coming in with their accompanying tank-farms, pipe-lines and people. In a short time the road between Saratoga and Batson Prairie was impassable, owing to the heavy machinery, pipe, and other oil field supplies that were being hauled over it. The drillers abandoned it and cut another road through the thicket. It rained steadily, and soon the new road was as bad as the old. There was nothing in that flat swampy country which would serve as a foundation for a road. As the mud got deeper and deeper, the major oil companies started to make a corduroy road by cutting down small trees and laying the trunks side by side.

I thought this an excellent road, but not for long. It was so narrow that it was impossible for two wagons to pass. A man on horseback could not pass a wagon without getting off in the mud, and the heavy wagons would break down and have to be unloaded. When this happened, the road would be blocked for hours. A heavy boiler often would cave in a wagon, then corduroy road and all would go down into the mud.

One day, when a group of young surveyors came into Saratoga, we learned they had come to survey the place for a branch line of the railroad into the oil field. After they had finished and located their site, we learned that the station was to be two miles from the old Hotel Saratoga, where most of us had located our places of business. Some time elapsed before we heard anything more from the railroad. We had almost forgotten about it in the mad rush in which we lived. Then news came to Saratoga that great crews of men were at work clearing away the trees and brush for the station, siding, and tracks.

People began to buy lots and build near the station. It was then discovered that there was no suitable place near the railroad to build the town. The lots were abandoned and the town was started in a man's little cornfield, which was in a small clearing, halfway between old Saratoga and the station. There was a mad scramble for the best locations in the town. Carpenters, near-carpenters, mule-skinners, and all those who could drive a nail or handle a saw, were pressed into service to build the new town. The town site was laid out with one long main street running through its center. On both sides of this street were the business houses. On two side streets were built the hotels, residences, and the numerous red-light houses.

I inveigled the owner of the town-site to build me a drug store, office, operating room, and bedroom in the center of this new town of Saratoga. This location was in the center of the town. After he had built my office and drug store, I persuaded him to bring over the post-office, which, up to that time, had been in his house, and put it in my drug store. Thus I had my office, drug store, sleeping quarters, and the post-office at my finger tips. Two large saloons on each side of me and one on each corner of the opposite side of the street, made it possible for me to reach the injured frequenters of these places without any trouble. Other doctors and drug stores came in, but I had the best location and had the reputation of arriving more quickly at a call than all others. I was also the physician for the Santa Fe Railroad which had come into the field.

By the time the railroad was ready to operate, we had the town laid out. Business houses, saloons, gambling joints, and houses of ill repute all were doing business on a big scale. Few of the saloons and gambling houses, and none of the red-light houses had front doors; so they were ready for business at all hours without the inconvenience to customers of opening and closing doors.

Gamblers, saloon-men, gun-men, pimps, and prostitutes crowded into the new town to get their share of the "pay day" spending. With the increasing number of oil companies these "pay days" were growing in number and size, and the residence district grew also. Men began to bring in their families and establish their homes. Many of the old settlers, who had lived for years in the Big Thicket, found themselves rich beyond their wildest imagination from oil under their lands. These soon moved to town and dressed up like advertising models for clothing stores. Those who had not reaped a harvest of gold from gushers and wells on their land, were working for companies and receiving fabulous wages and big bonuses for speed.

At first the dances were held in a large tent, but later a hall over a store was rented for such entertainment. I was always a guest at these dances in the hall, but in order to be present and still care for my practice, I used to keep my horse saddled and my emergency bag tied to it. I had my reputation for speediness in answering calls to maintain. The story became popular that I could get to a case in a saloon, gambling house, place of ill repute, or my office, dress the bruised and beaten person, and get back to a dance in time for the next number!

One night a man ran into the dance hall, with the name and number of a well where there had been an accident, and asked me to go there immediately. He started back to the well and I ran for my horse. I passed him on the road and was at the rig where the accident had occurred long before he got there. In drilling oil wells one part of the work is to let pipe down and pull it up with heavy machinery. A large hook is dropped down from the top of the derrick, and a helper fastens this hook into a gadget around the end of the pipe that is to be pulled up out of the well. In those days the man who operated this hook had to use speed and accuracy, for the hook came down like a shot and hardly stopped before it started back up at the same speed and, in that moment of pause, the helper had to make the connection or it was just too bad for him.

The man who had been injured at the well was the one who operated this hook. He was supposed to have fastened the hook into the ring on the pipe. Instead, his arm was caught in the hook. Up went the hook, hoisting the man in place of the pipe. Going up so fast without a load it started spinning rapidly, swinging the man around and around as he went up through the derrick. Before the driller could signal the hoist man to lower the hook, it was well up toward the top. By the time he was down and untangled from the machinery, his arm was broken in several places, and he was badly cut and torn about the face and body, and one eye was completely closed.

When I arrived, he was lying in a tool shack. With his uninjured hand he was holding a cigarette. I examined him, counted the different places his arm was broken, looked at that eye, the cuts and torn places, then said to myself, "No more dancing for me tonight."

HIGH LIFE

My drug store was built upon stilts like the other houses. It was on the corner, which made it more convenient for the town hogs to get underneath to sleep. Night after night my druggist drove them away and complained to the owners, but no attention was paid to his complaints. The next night the hogs would be back in their chosen quarters and, getting no relief from our roomers under the house, my druggist and I decided to take the matter into our own hands.

One bright day we fixed a couple of water guns that would squirt liquid with considerable force across the drug store. That afternoon the hogs, as usual, strolled under the drug store and were soon sleeping soundly. Across the street a group of gamblers and pimps were sitting on a pile of lumber talking and planning how they were going to skin the rough necks and drillers that night at the gaming tables.

Soon the store was echoing with the grunts and snores of my unwanted hog roomers under the house. Feeling that the time had come to do something about my tenants, my druggist and I filled our guns with "high life," went out the side door, knelt down on the ground close to the hogs and sprayed them. Then we retreated into the store as quickly as possible to wait for the show.

In a few minutes it started. When the "high life" had had time to take effect, it seemed to me that the drug store had been hit from below by an over-sized earthquake. I never knew before that there was so much speed in hogs. Down the street they went, grunting and squealing and making as much noise as a gusher. In their frenzied rush they did not attempt to stay in the road but, spread in all directions.

Before the gamblers and pimps realized what had happened, they were thrown in all directions. The hogs played no favorites, but took gamblers, whores, dogs, or children in their marathon race.

Soon the streets were full of amazed onlookers, for they had never before seen hogs act in such a way. A hog would stop, turn round and round, squeal, lie down, jump up, rub itself against buildings, and act as if it were crazy. Then, with a squeal, off it would tear trying to find relief.

After dusting themselves off, some of the gamblers held a conference and decided that all this commotion had started under my store. Ambling across the street, they asked my druggist what he had done. He feigned such surprise and innocence, however, that his questioners were unable to decide whether the druggist was telling them the truth or that they were being baited and by a "guy who didn't have no more sense than to work for his living."

A few days later one of the gamblers came into the drug store and whispered to the druggist and me that he wanted to speak to us privately. We took him back into my office. After the door was shut, the gambler told us that he wanted to buy some of the stuff that we had put on those hogs the other day.

When my druggist asked what he wanted to do with it, the gambler answered, "My old friend from up in the Big Thicket is in town again with all his family. Come here to the window and I'll show you."

Looking out of the window, we saw across the street an old wagon that looked as if it had been dragged out of the junk yard. Two horses, so poor we could count their ribs, were standing with their heads drooping half-way to the ground, sound asleep. Coming out of the saloon, in front of which the horses were standing, was an old man, thin, tall, stoop-shouldered, with long, shaggy, gray hair, drooping moustache, and about a four-year growth of beard. He was wearing an old black, slouch-hat, a ragged, red shirt, torn, blue overalls and worn-out, run-down boots.

Pointing to the old man, the gambler said, "Do you see the gentleman emerging from the palace of booze? Well, when that old son-of-a-bitch gets any money he comes to that saloon and stays there until it is all gone. He is the proud owner of those fine horses, that wagon, and all those beautiful animals under it."

Lying on the ground under the wagon was a pack of twelve or fifteen poor old hounds.

The gambler continued, "This owner declares that bunch of animals is the fastest in the Big Thicket. They can catch a bear, deer, hog, or anything that old fellow starts them after. I want to know whether or not it is true. I know that if you will just give me some of that stuff you put on those hogs the other day, I will see how fast they can run."

We gave him the bottle of high life. He took it and went across the street. Walking up to the old gentleman who was leaning against his wagon, he said, "Hello, Pop! How are you today?"

In a few minutes one old hound got up, scratched an ear with a hind foot, and tried to rub something off his back. He turned around two or three times, made a dash under the wagon, ran around the horses, let out a howl, and ran leaping down the street, howling louder with every leap. About that time two more hounds started acting the same way. By this time the old man was getting extremely excited about his hounds' actions, and we could see by his gestures that the gambler was trying to help him figure out what was the matter with his dogs. Each time the old man would turn away to talk to someone else about his hounds' peculiar actions, the gambler would pour high life on another dog.

In a few minutes up it would jump, start howling, run around the wagon, the horses, over to the old man and, with long ears flapping in the breeze, break for the jungle. This kept up until there was not a dog left.

The high life had been so successful with the hogs and hounds that Pinkey Pete, the bartender next door to my drug store, came into my office a few; days later and wanted a quart of "that stuff" my druggist had put on the hogs. I told him he was crazy; that a quart of that stuff would make the whole town take to the jungle. After much discussion as to the merits of a quart of it, he agreed to take a smaller amount, and my druggist sold him a little bottle full of it. After the bottle was wrapped, he said, "You know that son-of-a-bitch of Pug Mulligan? I don't want to kill him, but I'm a-goin' a see that he's run clean out of this town. I don't want to beat the damned bastard up, and I don't want to kill him, so I'm a-goin' to put some of this stuff on him. It'll fix him."

I tried to dissuade him, but he would not listen to me. That afternoon the saloon next door was full. The games were in full swing when Pug entered to get a drink and talk to the boys.

The feud between Pinky Pete, the bartender, and Pug Mulligan was one of long standing. Several times in the past they had tried to settle it with their fists. But the two were so evenly matched that neither one could whip the other. Both the men were fair minded and neither one wanted to kill the other, but everyone knew that some day the quarrel had to be settled.

Pinky Pete had just put his bottle of high life on the shelf where he kept his bottles and decanters when he saw his enemy walk into the saloon. Turning around he watched Pug for a moment, to see what he was going to do. Pug walked over to a table where a poker game was going on and stopped to watch it. The table was directly in front of the bar. As Pug stood watching the players, Pinky Pete poured a little of the high life into a small glass, reached across the bar, took careful aim, and threw it at him. Pug was too far away for much of it to get on him. Pinky Pete drew back his lips in a grin of gleeful anticipation and waited for the moment when the high life would begin to burn. He did not have long to wait. As he felt the tingle of the "stuff," Pug remembered what had happened to the dogs and the hounds. Wild with rage and swearing to kill Pinky Pete, he made a rush at him only to see the bartender poised with more of the liquid in a glass. As Pug did not have his gun, he made a break for the back door which he found shut and locked.

By this time the gamblers, drunks, and whores knew that something unusual was taking place. No guns were being drawn, no blows were being struck, just Pinky Pete chasing

Pug Mulligan around the saloon, with Pinky Pete holding a little glass in his hand. Pug Mulligan collided with a gambler who had just dumped his girl out of his lap, knocking the gambler down and tipping the girl over. By that time the gamblers and drunks, fearing what would happen if Pinky Pete should start throwing the high life at random, stampeded and began running over tables, chairs, and girls in a mad rush for the door. At last Pug found the front door and, as he went out of it, Pinky Pete threw the glass of high life at him. It not only hit Pug, but some of it sprayed the gamblers, pimps, girls and everybody else who happened to be near that door. Not satisfied with this "successful strike," Pinky Pete went out after Pug, and down the street they raced. For a block it was about a break away, but Pug was leading the race by a long margin. The high life helped him to keep up his speed. As Pinky Pete had nothing to help him run but his anger and, seeing how fleet of foot Pug had become, he realized that he never could catch up with him, and he returned to his saloon.

About three hours later he came over to my office and paid me for patching up the girls and gamblers who had gotten stepped on, knocked about, and burned in his and Pug's battle of high life.

SPOOKY GROUND

The oil field was expanding rapidly. Equipment was scarce; demands for wells to be drilled on leases swamped the contractors. In order to fill their orders, the contractors brought in antiquated boilers, using for fuel the crude oil from the wells. An apparatus was in use which would spray the oil against pieces of scrap iron in the boiler and convert it into a hot flame. The heat from this blaze made the power which ran the drilling rigs.

Sometimes, for some unknown reason, the oil would stop running through these apparatuses for a moment. When it stopped, gas would form in the fire-box. When the blaze started again, there was no use in calling the doctor. A few workmen with baskets to gather any pieces of bodies that they might find over the district was all that was necessary.

It seemed to me that these old boilers were set as close to the road as possible. Knowing the danger, I hated to ride past them. Often I was called to attend some person in charge of the operation of these boilers and I would have to stand in front or close to them as I prescribed. Needless to say, those patients received rapid treatment for their ailments.

At night the flare of the burning oil from these boilers lighting up the surroundings sent cold chills over me, for I knew the danger of explosions.

I had a patient in a tent near the old Saratoga Hotel. A contractor who had a couple of rigs running between the hotel and the tent where my patient lived had water lines and pipes spread out over the road where I had to cross to see my patient. He had cut down the trees and cleared away a place for his derrick-boiler, slush-pit and boiler house. One day as I started to call on my patient, I heard a blowing, hissing sound at the well. I stepped over the gas line and up to the derrick to talk with the driller a minute. I asked him about the strange noise. He replied that it was a little gas which had been encountered. I chatted a few minutes with him and went on to see my patient. When I returned, the noise had almost subsided.

A day or two later as I again started to see my patient, I heard the same roaring, hissing noise, which sounded as if that part of the country might be blowing up. Going close to the derrick, I saw the driller and all his men standing in deep conversation. As I stepped over the water line and started to where the men were standing, the ground under me began sinking. I took a few more steps, and it was worse. It seemed as if I were walking on a spring-board. I looked around at the giant pine trees that were standing near. They were standing erect, without moving, yet my sensation was that of walking across a carpet laid over springs. I never felt anything like that before. I had just come from a saloon where I had been treating a patient for D.T.'s, I had not had a drink, but I began to question my own sobriety.

I continued over this waving ground to where the men were standing. About the time I had reached them, mud and rocks started shooting up out of the well.

"Slim, what's the matter with the ground? Are you feeling what I feel? If you do, I think I am going far away from here at once," I said.

He laughed as he answered, "Well, Doc, she does feel like a rough sea, I admit. But, I wouldn't hurry away if I were you. The old girl is a bit excited but she'll calm down after a while."

"Sounds all right, Slim," I replied, "but I've been crossing this terra firma for some months and she never waved under me before. Your outfit just doesn't make sense."

He smiled, but his tone was grave as he told me that the thing didn't make sense to him nor did he like the way the ground was acting.

As I stood talking to the driller, the gas pressure became stronger and stronger. The mud and rocks were flung higher and higher and, as the rocks fell back to earth, they broke off large limbs of the great trees which stood in the path of their descent. I decided that I was in a big hurry to see my patient and rapidly departed.

The day after this well started to blow out, my father, one of the best men in the world, came to visit me. He had been a member of the Presbyterian Church for years and he lived his religion. Life was a serious thing to him, so serious, in fact, that he seldom laughed. Wanting to make his visit to me as entertaining and exciting as I could, I asked my father to go with me to see my patient. As we approached the well, I talked faster and louder of the wonders of the oil field. He listened attentively, but did not seem to be deeply impressed with my enthusiastic description.

Many people had gone over to the well to watch it blow out. As my father and I started toward it, we could hear the rocks hitting the trees as they came down. I told my father that we would go over and see the well, and we started across that springy ground. The first few steps I took I felt the ground begin to give under my feet. I smiled to myself and looked at my father's face. I could tell that he was not enjoying his walk. I stepped over a pipe line and I could hardly keep from running. It seemed as if the ground sank down a foot every step I took. I looked at my father as the ground waved and rolled under his feet. His face looked as if he had seen a ghost. I saw him glance here and there at the trees, and I knew that he was trying to reason out what was happening, but he did not say a word. I was anxious for my father to say something about the ground so that I could suggest that we go no closer to the well.

Just then the well roared louder than ever, and a shower of large rocks hit the ground directly in front of us. I glanced at my father, but he kept walking over that ground without saying a word. It felt as if I were stepping on springs without any cover on them, and the sensation was so terrifying that I felt it would be I who would have to call it quits. Just then the driller called to me not to come that way, but to go around where he and the people were standing. A look of relief passed over my father's face, but it did not compare with the feeling of relief I experienced.

When we reached the place where the driller was standing, I introduced my father to him, and asked him what was happening to the ground and the well. He told me it was the worst case of gas he had ever encountered and that he did not know what to expect. He told my father there was so much gas near the surface of the ground that it was causing the ground to move. Then he asked my father if he had noticed the ground's moving under him. He replied with only a simple, "Yes."

My father was a man of very few words, but this experience of walking on springy ground and roaring, hissing oil wells blowing mud and rocks hundreds of feet into the air, almost caused him to become altogether silent. The kindly but grave dignity with which my father had met all problems in life, had often made me wonder whether he could be shocked out of that calmness. The moving ground had not shaken it, but I thought I had one more opportunity to try.

The following night, which was Saturday, was my busiest night, for on that night people came from all over the Big Thicket to pay me, bring me word regarding patients, or to be treated themselves. Smiling to myself at my little plan, I told my father that night to make himself at home in the office and wait until I got through with my work. Later we would walk on the street and look for a man I wanted to see. He told me to go ahead with my work. I finished my work and we started out. We went down the street about two blocks, then back, where we came to the largest saloon and gambling house in town, located across the street in front of my drug store. I suggested that we go in there to see if I could find the man I was looking for.

The saloon was brilliantly lighted and crowded with as many people as could pack themselves into both the saloon and gambling room. It seemed as though the place was usually full of men and prostitutes, and all of them were full of squirrel whiskey. This was what I wanted my father to see. Back of the long bar was a mirror, which ran the whole length of the bar. On this mirror were painted the forms of women in their birthday suits. A dozen bartenders were dishing out bad drinks as fast as they could to a crowd of men and women lined up in front of the bar. Many of them were so drunk that they could not stand up without holding on to the bar. But they were still drinking, and the drunker they got, the more thoroughly the women went through the men's pockets as they embraced them.

The men and girls were talking, singing, cursing, quarreling and crying. I noticed my father's face set into a disapproving look as we pushed our way through this motley crowd back to the gambling room. It was a large room filled with all kinds of gambling paraphernalia, where men and women sat playing under the brilliant lights. The men were in different states of drunkenness. As large sums of money were lost, violent oaths and curses rent the air. Some of the girls were begging the men for more money to try their luck again. Some men sat at tables drinking with the girls who had on just enough clothes to make a fighting suit for a baby humming-bird.

My father started talking to himself like a sheep-herder. I could not tell what he said, but from the disgusted look on his face, I could tell that it was not complimentary to his surroundings. I thought that I had better hurry my joke on him before he left the place. Telling him that I must look in another part of the room, I slipped away and stood where I could watch him without his seeing me.

When I left him, a girl who looked old enough to be my grandmother began walking up to my father. Her hair was hanging around her shoulders. She had a wrinkled, painted face that looked like a topographic map. Practically nude and reeling with drink, she leaned toward him and looked at him with blood-shot eyes. In a whiskey-soaked voice she said, "Darling, don't you want to go home with me?"

Without speaking, he began backing away from that old girl as if she might be dynamite. I could see by the wild glances he was giving around the room that he was trying to locate me. Finally he started for the door as if he were fleeing for his life. Choking with laughter, I followed behind him, but keeping well behind and out of his sight. He got to the street door and left that place in a hurry. In a few minutes I found him waiting for me on the street corner.

Trying to keep my face straight, I apologized for having lost him in the gambling room. He looked at me with the same expression I had seen on his face when he led me, as a little boy to the wood-shed for a conference, and said, "Son, I would rather you would not stay in such a place as this." My father stayed a few days longer but, becoming restive, he left for home.

Three days later the well again started blowing out, but this time with the effect of an earthquake. The derrick man was up nearly at the top of the derrick when, as he said later, he thought that he felt it move. He was not quite sure whether it was the derrick moving or the effect of last night's squirrel-whiskey. As he was trying to make up his mind which it was, the derrick moved perceptibly to one side. The driller and his helpers started to leave the derrick on the run. The derrick man did not wait to come down the ladder, but used the crossbeams of the derrick which are about ten feet apart. He said that he came off that derrick like a flying squirrel, dropping from crossbeam to crossbeam and hit the ground running to the driller and the crew over to one side. Suddenly the ground seemed to rise like a great wave and sink back, taking with it the derrick. As it settled down, practically all the derrick sank with it, leaving only the extreme upper part above the ground.

Another rig in this same part of the field struck gas that would burn. Realizing the danger, the crew took every precaution to guard the well from exploding. One day a gentleman from a nearby city came out to see the oil fields and included this well in his tour. The driller had just finished telling him how inflammable the gas was and that they were prohibiting anyone from smoking around it. The man listened gravely to all the driller said, took his cigar from his mouth, and discovered that it was unlighted. He struck a match before anyone could stop him, the gas caught fire, and when they finally got the fire under control, part of that field was destroyed, and the injured workers who were not at the undertaker's filled my office to standing room only.

HAIL! HAIL! THE GANG'S ALL HERE!

One night I was called to one of the houses of ill repute. Before I arrived, I could hear singing, cursing, and crying all mingled together. I was met at the front door by the land lady's pimp. He calmly explained that he and his woman had had a fight and that he had "beaten hell out of her."

I had been called to fights at these houses often to repair the girls, and I thought that I'd find only the customary blackened eyes. The pimp took me down a hall which led to the back of the house. There in the little dirty kitchen, sitting on top of a small flat ice box, was his "woman."

She was a blousy, fat, sandy-blonde. She still had on what looked like the remains of some panties, and one stocking dangled over her foot. Outside of these remnants of clothing she could have posed as a little the-worse-for-wear model of a bulging and sagging "September Morn." Against each eye she was holding a large, raw steak. Her face was cut and blood was streaming from it and her nose and running down her neck, breast, and belly.

I looked around to see whether I could find anyone to give her a bath, for covered with blood as she was, I could not tell where to start patching her up. But her pimp, having done his manly and noble duty of calling a doctor for her, had left her and gone back to the saloon. There she sat on the ice box, a fit candidate for a nudist colony, cursing her pimp, crying, and wishing she were dead.

I looked around the kitchen for hot water, but I found neither hot water nor fire in the stove. Hearing raucous singing in another room, I went into it for help, only to find it filled with drunken men and women trying to dance and sing. They greeted me with shouts of welcome and begged me to come in and join them so that they could drink to my health. Both men and women were in all states of undress. They were the drunkest crowd I had yet seen in the oil field. I knew that I could not expect any help from them, so I left them to their debauchery and went back to the kitchen.

The patient was still sitting on the ice box holding her raw steaks to her eyes. Tears and blood were streaming down her cheeks, and through her cracked, swollen lips there would occasionally escape a vicious name, as she remembered what her recent fond assailant had done to her.

On a small jumbled shelf in the kitchen I found a small alcohol heater. Lighting it, I heated some water and got the patient to her room and started washing off the blood. I had almost finished dressing her wounds when, from the drunks in the other room, I heard a scream. Leaving my patient, I ran out into the hall to see what had happened. A man clothed in only part of his underclothes was dashing out of the front door, closely followed by a fat woman in her night dress and slippers. The man had been on a long drunken spree and had suddenly developed delirium tremens. He was making a dash for the brush, his woman close behind him trying to get him to come back to the house. The other drunks had followed them to see the fun. Finding that it was nothing serious, I went back to my patient, finished treating her, and left her and the drunks with what they called a good time.

After the railroad arrived in Saratoga, a lumber company put up one of the biggest sawmills in the district, three miles out of town. To assure the protection of their workmen's pure minds from being defiled by the flaunting of evil around them, the company bought a large tract of land around the mill and would not permit saloons, prostitutes, or gambling houses on the place. When the gamblers, saloon men, and prostitutes learned of this decree, they almost had heart failure, realizing what a big pay roll was turned loose each Saturday night without their having opportunity to share it.

Mac decided to do something about it. He went up to the lumber company's sawmill and picked out a piece of ground near it. This was located just outside the sawmill's property. There he built a saloon and gambling house.

The place had not been operating long before some of the sawmill boys started to show the oil field boys what it meant to be tough. So many people were killed there that the undertaker had to work overtime. It soon had such a bad reputation that the authorities had to send out a special deputy sheriff from Saratoga to keep some semblance of order.

One Saturday night, after the sheriff arrived, I was called to a confinement case at the sawmill. At that time I was having so many confinement cases that the saloon men and gamblers called me the fisherman. My patient was delivered about two o'clock in the morning and I started home. I had to pass by this gambling place. As I got close to it, I heard cursing, singing, women screaming, fighting, and laughter. I decided to see what the place looked like on Saturday night. Tying my bag to the horn of my saddle, I started up to the place from the side. The saloon was located at the front of the building, the gambling place in the rear. I was still outside when the owner came out of the saloon and started around to the gambling room on the side where I was approaching. He had a large pistol in his hand. He stopped, raised his gun, and called out, "Who is there?"

"Turn that gun the other way," I answered.

He recognized my voice and replied, "Doctor, what in hell are you doing out here this time of the night? Come here."

He sounded as if it were imperative, and I walked rapidly over to where he stood.

"Don't you know the meanest set of men and women in the whole world are in my place tonight?" he said. "Come in with me, but stay close to me, I want to show you something."

We entered the gambling place, which was a long, wide room filled with more gambling paraphernalia than I had ever seen. The room was crowded with a motley throng of Negroes, Mexicans, Americans, and foreigners. The Mexican women had long, thin knives stuck in their hair or belts. Negro wenches held razors. Men with pistols strapped on their hips were being embraced by the women. They were without doubt the toughest, hardest-looking bunch of crooks I had ever seen. I had seen tough men in the West and in other parts of Texas, but I had never seen such a crowd of them as I was looking at in that saloon.

The gambler turned to me and said, "Doctor, what do you think of my guests?" Without waiting for me to reply, he continued, "I have gambled and run gambling houses in New York, Mexico, Central and South America, and the Klondike, but for downright mean cut-throats I have never seen anything like this. Look them over. I have seen individual sons-of-bitches and even two or three together, but never before have I seen sons-of-bitches in droves like this."

While he was speaking, a tall, muscular, blonde man, showing his Germanic origin, stepped up to the dice table. Little, cold, pale blue eyes, peered expressionless from beneath sandy eyelashes. Thick, cruel, sensuous lips held an unlighted, half-chewed cigar. He slipped a great, square-fingered hand into his pocket and took out a roll of one-hundred dollar bills. Peeling off one of them he threw it on the table, picked up the dice, threw them, and won.

"Watch that son-of-a-bitch," whispered the gambler.

The gambling attendant threw a hundred dollar bill on top of the German's. He let it lie there, reached for the dice, shot again and won. The attendant threw down two hundred dollar bills. Without noticing them, the German reached for the dice, shot, and won. The attendant laid down four hundred bills. Again the German won. Reaching into the drawer for a roll of bills and counting out eight hundred dollars, the attendant put them on the stack of money on the table. By this time the other gamblers in the room had quit playing to watch the German. The German again reached for the dice.

I said to the proprietor of the gambling house, "Mac, won't that guy break the bank?"

The gambler laughed and replied, "No, I have a bale of that stuff. I won't need to lay much more down. And the attendant will rake it all back into the drawer."

The German continued to shoot dice and win without picking up the money, until there lay on the table more than six thousand dollars. By this time the table was crowded with onlookers. Then the German reached again for the dice, shot, and lost. The attendant calmly reached for the money, put it into the drawer and, without speaking, shoved it shut. The German walked over to another table and began playing another type of game.

Mac told me that the German played every Saturday night, but up to date his total loss to the gambling houses amounted to only a few hundred dollars. He confided to me that while often the players won, most of the gamblers lost. Were it not so, a gambling house could not stay in business.

He told me about some men in Beaumont who gambled in a little insignificant two-story frame building across from the Crosby Hotel. Only business men sat in that game. The stakes were oil lands, producing wells, and business.

POISON GAS

Days merged into weeks, weeks into months, and my bank account grew as my practice increased. One afternoon, just before dark, as I was preparing to leave my office, a telegram was handed to me. There being no telephone communication in Saratoga at that time, the telegraph served for all emergencies. This telegram was from one of the big oil companies in the field, asking me to come to Batson Prairie to attend a driller who had been gassed. I knew that it was an emergency case. Night was coming on, and the journey did not arouse my enthusiasm, for I knew that road. Since it was a matter of duty and must be done, I decided to start at once and ride fast so that I would have less riding in the dark.

Arriving at the shack, I found the driller lying on a cot, to all appearances, dead, his eyes open, lips parted, swollen, and dark as if burned with acid. It was with difficulty that I could find a pulse or detect any respiration. I worked with him until morning. At times through the night it seemed as though his heart would stop in spite of all that I could do. I gave him the medicine that I had developed and used so successfully with the gas cases in Saratoga, but he showed very little sign of life until after daylight next morning. I had been treating men at Saratoga for months and had seen them stay unconscious for a few hours and then recover, but this one was unconscious for more than twelve hours.

This case gave me a new idea on gas poisoning. At Saratoga, when these cases first began to appear, it was something new to me, and I immediately began to study them and talk to the old-time oil men, but none of them could give me any information on this form of gas poisoning. I searched medical books and journals, and delved back into my mind trying in vain to remember hearing of such cases at Medical School or in the hospitals. I wrote to the Dean of the Medical School where I studied medicine. He was a brother fraternity man and I knew that he would help me if he could. I described the gas cases to him and asked him what to do for my patients. "Damned if I know," was the terse information he contributed.

I had developed a medicine for the eyes of those who were gassed so badly that they had to stay in a dark room for several days. Also in my research work I had discovered something that eliminated the danger to the heart and lungs in gas cases. I thought I had this gas poisoning pretty well in hand, but this first Batson Prairie patient destroyed my satisfaction in my progress in medicine and gave me something more to think about. I therefore intensified my studies of gas. I did not have long to wait; for in a few days I was called to a case of another type of gas poisoning on which to try my new medicines.

My next gas patient was a young man whose eyes were bulging out around the colored parts, the whites of the eye lids almost completely hiding the iris. I gave him an emergency treatment and told him to come back later. I was hoping that the whites of his eyes would be normal when he returned, but they were not. I did not know what else to do, so I continued applying the medicine I had developed to counteract the effect of the gas on his eyes. In a few days he was cured, but I never saw another case of eye trouble like that one.

A few days after I had dismissed the patient with the bad eyes, another emergency call came from Batson Prairie. When I arrived, I found two girls and a young man gassed. They had gone to a hydrant for water and, while they were filling their buckets, a wave of poisonous gas had blown over them. They had fallen unconscious to the ground at the same time. The people who had seen them fall rushed over to them, but not one of the rescuers was gassed. The reason for this was that the gas had been blown away before they ran to rescue the fallen ones.

They carried the three gassed people to their nearby tents. One of the girls and the man were lying as if dead. Not a movement, no perceptible breathing, and scarcely any pulse.

But the other girl was flopping around over the bed like a chicken with its head chopped off. Two men were holding her down, and they worked all night in relays holding her on the bed. I worked all night to keep the heart and lungs of the one girl and man going and to calm the other girl, so that her excited condition would not overtax her heart. At the same time I gave all of them medicine to eliminate the poisoned condition. It was long after sun-up before any of them showed any signs of returning to consciousness. All three of them returned to normal within thirty minutes of each other.

There was something so sinister about this gas that I felt as if I were fighting against something intangible and phantom-like. Different gases from different fields would attack different parts of the body and affect the person in a different way. This gas was turning my hair white, for I was receiving calls at all hours of the day and night, from all the different fields.

One night, when I was returning to Saratoga from a call to Batson Prairie, I almost became its victim myself. I was riding alone when a wave of the poisonous gas struck me. I put the spurs to my horse and rode like mad, holding my breath as long as I could. I almost fell off my horse. But it gave me a scare which helped me to dig harder into medicine than ever to see whether or not anyone could supply information on gas poisoning.

A few days after I met that gas on the road, an emergency call came from Batson Prairie. A new well had come in during the night, with more poison gas. The wind had changed during the early morning and wafted the gas into the town. People, chickens, cattle, and horses were dropping dead by the score. The authorities sent out runners over the town awakening those who were still in bed. As the alarm spread, the streets were soon filled with men, women and children in day clothes and night dress, fleeing for their lives.

That was one time when no one turned back for anything but his children. Fleeing men would stop to pick up and drag to safety those who had fallen unconscious on the road. Possibly, before they reached the next block, one of the rescuing ones would fall, and the unconscious one would recover, and start dragging the person just overcome. Women, running a race with the "Old Man" and his scythe, dragged and pulled babies and children, their faces set and strained with the horror of the death they faced.

Many died in their sleep before the runners could awaken them. Chickens, horses, cattle and people lay dead in their homes and in the streets. In a short time after death had overtaken them, they were swollen to such proportions they were unrecognizable. Indeed Death walked abroad in Batson Prairie that tragic day, laying his icy hand on young and old alike.

THEY DIED WITH THEIR BOOTS ON

From the wealth of the oil field it was destined that many characters, both famous and infamous, were to be made. A family of brothers came into Saratoga, became millionaires, and one of them, in later years, went to the State Capitol of Texas as Governor. There also grew up in the oil fields an organization of gunmen and racketeers. The mounting pay rolls and freely circulating money attracted the toughest characters from all parts of the globe. These outlaws made it their business to prey on the "rough-necks" who were earning a great deal of money in the field. They would attack them on the road, as they staggered back from their drunken debauches, rob them and, if they put up any fight, beat them, or kill them, and toss their bodies into a shallow grave or the bayou. Many of the girls of ill fame were also their victims. Since they were making lots of money and no one cared enough to protect them, they fell prey to this killing robbing element.

The crime wave had become so desperate that the authorities sent a deputy sheriff to the district, a fearless man who had killed many men. The crooks were aware of his efforts to break up their organization and he became a marked man.

One Saturday night the leaders of this organization decided to hold up one of the saloons and gambling houses on the road to the sawmill. Someone had given the sheriff the information that these gangsters were going to make a raid on the saloon that night, but his pride and egotism caused him to make very little preparation for the raid.

About eleven o'clock, when the saloon was filled with drunken men and girls and the games in the gambling-house were at their height, three of the gangsters walked in the front door of the saloon. The sheriff was standing near the bar waiting for their appearance. When they saw the sheriff, they jerked out their guns and started shooting at him. At the first shots the customers, bartenders, and girls dropped to the floor, or ran crouching to the exits. As the sheriff saw the men draw their guns, he drew his and started shooting, killing one and wounding the other. Two of the gang, who had entered the back door of the gambling house when their three "pals" had entered the saloon, heard the shooting and ran into the saloon, drawing their pistols and shooting at the sheriff from behind. He reeled and fell. As he was falling, he aimed at a bandit who had just entered the front door of the saloon and killed him.

The two bandits who had entered the saloon from the gambling-room were still shooting at the sheriff as he hit the floor. He rolled over on the floor, raised himself on his elbow, blood flowing from his mouth from the bullet wounds in his lungs, took aim at the bandits with his pistol, shot one dead, and seriously wounded the other. Then with a convulsion running through his body, he fell back dead.

The prostitutes, thugs, gunmen, and gangsters in Batson Prairie finally became so terrible that the authorities sent in the Texas Rangers to keep order.

One night some fellows were walking down the streets. They had been partaking of too much liquid nourishment. As they passed a brilliantly lighted saloon, one of the drunks looked through the window of the saloon and saw the bartender dispensing drinks to the crowd. He stopped suddenly and said to his fellow drunk, "I believe I'll just kill that son-of-a-bitch," whipped out his gun and, before his companion could stop him, had shot the bartender dead. He had no reason for his act. Perhaps he was but proving to the world his right to self-expression and personal liberty.

After the Saratoga boom was well-developed, a family came in there and opened up a boarding house near the station. They had a slender, nice, intelligent-looking boy about fifteen years old. His mother was a fine, self-sacrificing woman, who was always trying to care for someone else. Her boarders consisted principally of rough-necks and gamblers. I soon noticed her boy staying around the saloons and gambling-joints, associating with the saloon men and gamblers. He never had a job, and never seemed to be seeking one, but he always seemed to have plenty of money. As he grew a little older, I noticed how mean and cruel his face was be coming, how cold and merciless were his light-blue eyes. He soon had a reputation in that oil-field as a fighter but he never used his fists, always a knife or a pistol. One night he shot a man. The man died, and the boy disappeared, leaving his mother heart-broken, for she had tried to help him to decent manhood. In a few months he again showed up at Batson Prairie, meaner than ever and quicker on the draw. He killed another man at Batson Prairie and soon became an important bully around the red light houses, saloons, and gambling dens. The pimps, saloon-men, and gamblers gave him a wide berth, and none of them would dispute his word. He grew more and more daring, and was soon boss of the thugs and crooks.

At about that time a new crowd of gangsters from the outside came to Batson Prairie with the idea of doing a wholesale business in crime. They wanted to make their leader head of the bad men and did not want to recognize this boy as their leader. None of them, however, was so quick on the draw as he, and he soon had the undisputed leadership over the bad men. He kept cutting notches on his gun until he had it heavily encrusted with them.

Suddenly he disappeared from Batson Prairie, and no one seemed to know why. He was gone for quite some time. One day he reappeared in Batson Prairie, as suddenly as he had disappeared. He was far tougher, harder, and meaner than ever. He started killing on a much larger scale than before, until even the peace officers had considerable respect for him. His reputation as a killer grew. He soon had a saloon and gambling house of his own and, with the various rackets he had on the side, he had the substantial advantage over the other bad men. Those who did not respect his power soon found how accurate and deadly his aim was. Most of them took him as a matter of course, for they were not yet ready to leave the oil fields, nor did they care to decorate his gun.

One day a man who appeared to be about thirty years of age, tall, slender, with straight black hair and icy grey eyes, that looked as if each one of them was tipped with a steel jacket from a pistol cartridge, came to Batson Prairie. He was plainly dressed, but not in the garb of a roughneck or gambler. He did not tell anyone his name, where he came from, or anything about his business. He soon became known merely as "Stranger," and to that name he made no comment, save genially to recognize it when so called.

He talked very little, did not seem to have anything special to do, anywhere to go, or be in any hurry to get there. He bought a shack, lived alone, frequented the saloons, and drank, but not with anyone else.

He was absolutely indifferent to the bullying demands of the Batson Prairie bad man who had come to be known in the oil fields as the "Bad Boy."

Bad Boy could not stand the silence and indifference of the Stranger, so he sent word to him to get out of town and get out quick, or he would kill him on sight. Stranger listened to the message and went on the even tenor of his way, just as he had been doing. The gamblers and some of the others who had taken a liking to Stranger tried to impress upon him the seriousness of Bad Boy's warning, but it made no impression on him.

One afternoon, as Stranger was going down Main Street in Batson Prairie, he saw Bad Boy coming up the opposite side of the street. His friends yelled at Stranger to run, and all of them scurried into the saloon. Paying no attention to the shouts of warning, Stranger kept walking down the street in the direction of Bad Boy. When Bad Boy came opposite the man, he turned and started to cross the street toward him. As he neared Stranger, he called him a vile name and at the same time, reached for his gun. The next instant Bad Boy was pitching forward in the street with three bullets in him, his unfired gun falling from his almost lifeless hand. Stranger walked over to where Bad Boy had fallen and stood looking down at him without a change of expression. Bad Boy rolled over, raised himself on his elbow, the blood gushing from his mouth and nose.

Stranger said quietly, "Get up, you son-of-a-bitch; I want to shoot you again."

The only answer from Batson Prairie's Bad Boy was a gasp as he fell back dead. Thus finished the ignominious career of one of the worst men in the oil fields, shot by the still unknown Stranger.

THE ART OF MANLY DEFENSE

I had many cases of malaria of the type that eats away the patient's resistance and keeps him down with slow fever for months. Although the patient might remain the same for weeks, the doctor was afraid not to keep calling on him. There was danger that the family might give him something to eat and then tell him, "Good-by," or that, in his extreme weakness, his heart would stop beating. With a dozen of these slow fever cases, emergencies, fights, confinements, and the prostitutes always needing to be patched up, a doctor was kept going day and night.

The attitude of the oil field toward life or death was clearly expressed by the nurse who attended a patient of mine with a severe case of fever. I was doing all I knew to do, but he was getting worse and worse. His fever kept climbing and climbing. I called in consultation all the practicing physicians in the district as well as some of the doctors who were in business there but not in active practice. No one seemed to be able to suggest anything that would aid him. I could not get a trained woman nurse, but a male nurse whom I had called on the case was very fine. One day the patient called the nurse and said, "Bill, I believe I am going to have to lay 'em down."

Without turning from fixing the medicine he was going to give him, the nurse said, "Ah! Hell, John, you ol' son-of-a-bitch, don't lay 'em down yet." But with all this strong advice not to "lay 'em down," he went ahead and did that very thing.

I had a young lady patient who had lived out in the Big Thicket all her life. She had contracted a long and bad case of typhoid fever. I told the old ignorant mother that under no circumstances was she to let her have anything to eat but the diet I had prescribed. About two days later, after I had practically dismissed the patient, an urgent call came to go to see her. When I arrived at the house, I looked at the unconscious girl lying on the bed, lips blue, eyes set, the death look on her face. I asked her mother what she had given her to eat. She began to cry and said that the girl's brother had killed a young, fat squirrel, and the girl was so hungry and had begged so hard for it that she had given her just a little bit. The "little bit" had signed the girl's death warrant.

As I was going over to Batson Prairie one morning on a call, I came to the Bayou, where I found another small town in the making. Some of the major oil companies had decided to build a tank-farm a short distance from the new crossing. This had all been done in the four days which had passed since I had last been to Batson Prairie. Several wagons were there, scrapers and tools had been unloaded, and men were busy clearing the ground and putting up tents. I knew that as soon as they had a few tents up the saloon-keepers, gamblers, and prostitutes would be there.

The company brought in more workmen and began building pipe-lines, tanks, and houses for their employees. Soon the roughest and worst toughs in all the oil fields were congregated at this point. Not long after the company had finished this new camp, the gun-men, saloon-keepers, gamblers, pimps, and prostitutes were settled there in their new homes. As the months passed, this new town gained the reputation of having the worst class of criminals in all the field.

A white man came into this new town and built about twenty shacks in a row. They were made out of palms with no floors, their furnishings consisting of one dirty cot, a washstand, and a chair. A door in front of the huts and a little window in the rear were all the openings the shacks had. When the shacks were finished, the owner left town for two weeks and, when he returned, he brought in the toughest Negro wenches anyone ever saw, one for each shack. He figured that with the tough element running the saloons and gambling houses, these wenches could get most of the Bayou payroll. They were not girls of easy morals; they simply did not have any morals. The only thing they did have was pure devil. They would commit any crime for fifty cents. Morning after morning white men's bodies would be found floating in the Bayou, victims of these wenches. The place had the reputation of being the filthiest, meanest, arid most hellish that had ever entered the oil field. But when that white man left the oil fields, he took out enough money to last him the remainder of his life.

One night I was hurriedly called to see a patient in this new town, I arrived at the Bayou just after dark. I had to go past the Negro prostitutes' houses. Whew! That place made my hair stand on end with fear as I hurried past it. The singing, cursing, and noise which was floating out on the air from those gambling shacks and saloons made one's heart turn sick.

Later Batson Prairie's houses of prostitution grew to be equally as bad. Just off the main street, in the thicket, were a group of these houses clustered around two old ramshackle, two-story houses, built at right angles to each other, and joined together at the back. This particular place was far worse than Hell's Half-acre. The two old houses had the regular saloons in front with gambling houses in the rear. The upstairs of both houses was divided into small rooms just large enough for a dresser, a bed, and a chair. Cut into the wall were small windows which let in a bit of light during the day. The only other light which entered the narrow, dismal halls running through these houses came from the smoking oil lamps.

When emergency calls came to me to go to these houses and I had to pass through those dark, rambling halls, I felt as though hands were reaching out to tap me on the head or choke me to death. Only the knowledge that the pimps, gamblers, and gunmen who lived in these places felt friendly toward me gave me the courage to answer the calls. Otherwise the largest fee they could have offered would not have tempted me to enter one of these houses.

It was in a saloon near these houses where two prostitutes, one white, the other a Negro wench, one day started a fight. The officers arrested both of them. Then they tried to decide what to do with them. While they were consulting the points of law of this particular case, one of the interested bystanders had a brilliant idea. He suggested to the officers that they let the girls fight it out, and the one who won the fight should go free. The girls thought that a just and splendid idea, and the officers thought it was an answer to their law problem.

The men marked off a ring in which the two women were to fight, stripped them to their waists, took the wench's razor away from her, and turned them loose. There were no ring rules; so it was a scratching, hair-pulling, biting, kicking, punching affair, with honors to the white girl. Whenever I had to pass the Bayou or be out at night, I rode with my pistol drawn covering anyone I met. Conditions were so bad that it was worth one's life to be out in that section after nightfall. My horse had a white spot in his forehead, and everybody knew him as my horse. As I would meet a person on the road, I would cover him with my pistol until we came abreast of each other. I would then see him slip his gun back into his belt, and I would put mine away as he would say, "Hello, Doc! Where the hell are you going this time of night?"

One of the Batson Prairie oil company's drillers became famous as a bully. His technique of bullying was backed up by his ability to fight. He was an expert driller and was always employed. Thus he worked in the day and fought in the saloons at night. Soon he had the reputation of being the best fist fighter in that region. And how he loved and defended his reputation! If any person showed signs of resentment to this driller's bullying, that person was in for a nice licking. For several months the bully carried all honors in his field, but I could not complain, for he was a splendid business-getter for me. I patched up many a one he had decorated with his fists.

A new company came in and brought their own crew and drillers with them. They cleared a place, erected a derrick, and started work.

After the day's work the new company's crew and drillers would come to the saloons and gambling houses. Among the new crew of drillers was a tall, angular man, who looked as though if he got his own business attended to he would be satisfied. The bully started in to let these new men know who was boss of that region. He bullied the tall redhead several times, but the latter never replied to anything he said. So the bully decided that he had the fellow afraid of him and would give him a working over.

One Saturday night one of the popular saloons was full of men. The bully, swaggering and boasting, was there with his friends. Presently the tall redhead came in alone. The bully said something to Redhead which he did not like and, for the first time he answered the bully. The words had no more than passed the redhead's lips than the bully went into action to impress on the fellow as quickly as possible that he was to be respected. It was a straight fist fight, just the type the bully lived for. But Redhead surprised the bully, for he did not take the count as quickly as others had been doing.

One thing which the bully never permitted on his pro grams was for another to hit him in the face. As the bull rushed into the fight, Redhead whammed him on the nose, and the blood poured out of it in quantities.

They fought and fought, neither of them yielding in the evenly-matched fight. Finally, both of them began to tire. Blood was dripping from the cuts on their swollen and bruised faces, when suddenly Redhead made a nice pass and pasted the bully a smack in the left eye. As the bully started for the floor, one of his friends decided that it was time for him to take a hand in the fight and stepped up to take a poke at Redhead. Just then a voice rang through the room.

"I'll kill the first son-of-a-bitch who touches either one of them."

It was the bartender who had been watching the fight. He had stepped up on the bar and there he stood above the crowd, a slender, nice-looking fellow, in his hand an old, long, black pistol which he waved slowly over the heads of the crowd. At his command all eyes, including the bully's friend looked up. They knew from those cold, steel-gray eyes that whoever started to help the bully was as good as dead as soon as he made the move. Somehow the bully's friend lost all desire to save his laurels.

The interruption gave a short respite to the combatants. When the bully learned that there was to be no aid granted, he started the fight again. On they fought until they fell exhausted to the floor, still making futile passes at each other as they lay there. The bartender finally called it a draw. I was then called upon to patch up their faces and bruises.

On another Sunday morning one of the saloons was filled with men, drinking, swearing, and gambling. In front of the bar stood a rough-neck with all the squirrel whiskey he could hold. The more squirrel whiskey he drank, the louder he boasted of his ability to lick any son-of-a-bitch in town. He was so persuaded of his prowess that he kept punctuating his sentences by thumping the bar with his fist to impress on his audience the force of his blows. Another man stood by him, leaning with his back against the bar, his heel hooked in the rail. He had been drinking also but was not so drunk as the boasting battler.

Suddenly the boasting battler turned around and said something to the other man, who slowly took his heel off the rail and, without turning round, straightened his arm out on the bar, and let drive, without saying a word. The punch caught the battling boaster on the side of his head, shot him neatly through the window of the saloon, and deposited him in the street. So, I had another to patch up.

CHRISTMAS IN THE OIL FIELDS

Before the oil field came in to turn the "Big Thicket" into a mad-house, the old settlers had a little church which they attended. After the oil field came in and the money began flowing, many of the youngsters belonging to the old settlers decided to take the "broad path" and try the evils that were being introduced to them.

In the beginning of the oil field scramble, one of the major oil companies had sent an old gentleman into Saratoga as their manager. He was a cultured, highly-educated man and formerly a minister. Whiskey was an abomination to him, and he did not tolerate anyone who used it. He made a ruling for his workmen that any one of them who got drunk was automatically discharged.

The first week he started I held my breath, for I knew the type of men he was employing. Saturday night came, and he turned loose a large payroll. Monday morning every man reported for duty. The next week all his men stayed as sober as judges. Payday came, and another big pay-roll was turned loose. Monday all the crew and drillers reported for duty, not a drunk among them. By that time I was wondering whether I had misjudged these men and whether only a firm hand was needed to keep them straight. The whole field, by now, was wondering how long this reformation was going to last.

One night, however, his whole outfit broke rank, and the saloons, gambling houses, as well as the prostitutes, felt the golden rain of the money, which had been restrained too long in the pockets of the drillers and rough-necks. The old manager made good his word. Every man who had been drunk was not permitted to come back on the job.

One husky rough-neck, whose drunk lasted from Saturday until Tuesday, reported for work on Wednesday. The manager told him that he was fired, and that he was to go to the office and get his money. Instead of going to the office for his money, he went to the saloon and got drunk again. He stayed drunk until his money gave out, and then he remembered about his wages and decided that he would go and get them from the company. He came into my drug store on his way to the oil company's office, which was just across the street. He told the druggist he was going over to collect his wages. He was then so drunk that he was barely able to walk. Knowing the manager's hatred of drink and the strict law he had enforced with his men, I went to the window to see what would happen.

The popular song called, "Show Me The Way To Go Home, Babe," was being whistled on every side in the oil field. The drunk zigzagged across the street. Suddenly he broke out singing this song in a loud, but drunken voice. After much effort he finally reached the opposite side of the street. A little fence, with a closed gate, barred admittance to the office. The drunk tried to open that gate without success. I was jittery, watching him fumbling with its fastening. Suddenly his hand hit the latch and he opened the gate and staggered on to the narrow gallery running across the front of the office.

The manager arose and went to the door of the office as the man made for the door and asked him how he dared to come on the company's property in such a drunken state. The man looked at the manager as he angrily told him about the rules of the company. When the manager had ceased speaking, the drunk went Grand-Opera and started singing in a loud voice which could be heard a block away, "Write me out a pension for the rest of my life, And show me the way to go home." That was the final straw. The manager showed him how to go home, right off the porch and through the gate, without a pension for the remainder of his life.

It was this dignified, highly-cultured, ex-minister, manager of the oil company, who officiated as minister at the little church. A few of the old settlers, the manager, and I attended the services. The old settlers soon found out how much excitement and pleasure money could buy them, and they left the church for the saloons and gambling houses.

Soon it was only the preacher and I who attended services at the little church. We called a Board Meeting consisting of the two of us and decided that if we moved the church into town and built a nice building, maybe some of the new oil field residents would attend.

As the old settlers were now fabulously wealthy from their oil lands, it was no trouble to get money for the new church. It was completed by Christmas. Such a crowd as there was on the streets. Men, women, children, pimps, gamblers, thugs, prostitutes, oil field workers, lease owners, contractors, foreigners from all parts of the globe, drifters, and adventurers; all laughing, happy in the mellowness of Christmas Eve.

The night was clear and bright with stars. In the church, glittering with Christmas decorations and tinsel, stood the largest tree which would fit into the corner. Showy, rich, and expensive presents lay under the tree. Every one there had an enjoyable time, and afterwards all went to the Christmas Eve dance at the hall.

The people who had lived in the "Big Thicket" before the oil well boom had never known such finery and gaiety existed in the world until the past few months, when wealth poured into their hands so fast they could spend only a fractional part of it. They seemed dazed with it all. Their sons and daughters did not have this trouble, but rapidly learned how to dispense with the golden flow.

Christmas morning came, and the whole town seemed to be drunk. The Saratoga Hotel served a late Christmas breakfast, for the proprietor was afraid that by noon his guests would not be able to sit up and eat an elaborate dinner. He served breakfast at eleven o'clock. To most of the guests partaking of the breakfast, it meant more liquid nourishment, with the proprietor leading in the partaking. They could not see any reason for eating food when there was so much to drink. I left the breakfast in disgust and went to my office.

As I neared my drug store, a large crowd was standing on the corner cheering and seemingly well entertained. As I drew nearer, I saw in the center of the crowd two big husky rough-necks trying to settle their Christmas differences with punches that sounded as if a mule were kicking a barn door. I watched them a few minutes and, as I saw the blood flowing freely, I knew that it was time to go to my office and get plenty of hot water ready. I was none too soon, for shortly I was patching cuts, stopping hemorrhages, putting lotions on bruises, and trying to get the swelling down out of punched eyes. By dinner time, sixteen fights had taken place within two blocks of my office. The patients were coming so rapidly that I could not attend to them fast enough. I pressed into service some helpers so that I could clear the office more quickly and give room to those coming in. The victors and defeated all needed working over. As they sat side by side in my office waiting their turns to be treated they promised one another what they were going to do as soon as they could.

I had the office fairly well cleared when a man was led in with one eye swollen shut and a great gash under the other from which blood was flowing. His nose was smashed, and he was spitting blood and teeth. I started on him and was getting along very well when someone in the drug store cried, "Fight!" I was wondering how I was going to get away from my patient long enough to see it. I looked at one eye tightly closed and thought that if I could get him to hold a pledget of cotton over the other eye with the gash under it, I could see the fight and attend his wounds later. I picked up a piece of cotton as big as my fist, dabbed it in a solution, put it over his eye, and told him to hold it there a while. When I was sure that he could not see, I ran to the porch of my drug store.

Directly in front of the drug store two men were fighting like tigers. One would knock the other down, wait for him to get up, then they would start all over again. The crowd was cheering them wildly. Around and around they went, until they had to rest from sheer exhaustion. When the crowd saw that they could not fight to a finish, they lost interest and drifted back into the saloons.

I thought that I would go back to my patient when I heard a voice on the other side of the post against which I had been leaning watching the fight say, "Well, I'll, be damned."

I looked around and there leaning against the post stood my patient. He had pulled the cotton down from his eye just far enough to look over it at the fight. When he saw that the fight was finished, he turned to me and said, "Well, Doc, let's get back to our business."

We went back into the office. I finished him up and soon had him on the street all bandaged up, with one eye sticking out, looking for trouble.

THE BAYOU

At twilight, one evening, as I was on my way to Batson Prairie, a wet "norther" started, and the chill of that rain and wind seemed to pierce one through and through. The holes in the road were filled with water, and the mud was deep. As I rode on, I passed wagon after wagon loaded with heavy machinery, sunk in the mud down to the hubs of the wheels. The mule-skinners were lashing and cursing their rearing and plunging mules and oxen.

A few hundred yards before I came to the crossing of the bayou, a wagon was stopped on the road. I rode around it and found another wagon was stopped in front of it. At the bayou crossing, I could hear shouting, cursing, swearing, and the singing of the long whips the mule-skinners cracked over the backs of their teams. Urging my horse on, I came to a place where a large clearing had been made on both sides of the road, where it crossed the bayou. Wagon after wagon stood in the road, their drivers cursing and urging their teams forward.

In the bayou a big wagon with an old boiler on it had sunk down into the mud and water. It had evidently been there for some time. The man who was the driver of the team had cut down trees and, with long pieces of timber and poles, he and his helpers were trying to prize the sunken wagon out of the mud and water. Some of the drivers of the other wagons had brought their mules and hitched them in front of those which were pulling the wagon. The mule-skinners were cursing the cold and rain, which, by now, had changed to sleet and fleecy flakes of snow. Soon, over the scene, a white whirling snow began falling. It was such an exciting scene that I rode up on the bank of the bayou and stopped my horse for a better view.

A provisional road had been cut around the wagon where the boiler was stuck, and wagons were trying to crossover this new road. But the men who were trying to get the wagon out of the mud were taking up so much room in the road and bayou and making so much noise, that the other mule-skinners could not coax their mules into the water. They were all yelling and swearing at the mules and at one another. Soon from the Batson Prairie direction appeared the contractors, who were in a hurry for their machinery and were worrying about the delay. As they joined the crowd, they began to curse the men with the boiler. The mule-skinners finally succeeded in getting their mules and wagons into the bayou but, as they tried to urge them around the wagon, the mud, slush, and water churned in dark eddies around the legs and bellies of the plunging mules and pulled the wagons deeper into the mud which held them. The long whips sang through the air to lay open the sides and flanks of the straining animals and color the brown water with blood, but the wagons only sank deeper into the mud.

While I was watching the scene, a mule, in its rearing and plunging, slipped and fell. The driver, cursing and swearing in a frenzy of rage, repeatedly slashed it with his long whip until its side and flank were streaming with blood. Just then a deputy sheriff rode up, watched the skinner for a moment; then got down off his horse, walked over to the skinner, cursed him, and ordered him to stop slashing the mule. The mule-skinner stepped back from the deputy the length of his whip and answered by cracking the deputy in the face with it, cutting away part of his face. The officer whipped out his pistol and shot the mule-skinner dead.

In contrast to this, one of the most weird and beautiful scenes I had ever seen was at the bayou. I was called one night to Batson Prairie to see a patient. As I rode along, suddenly it seemed as if the whole Thicket must be burning up. I looked ahead, but could see nothing. The light grew brighter, and a crackling sound, as if a forest were burning, sounded through the night. I could see a wide band of flame running along the ground and leaping high into the trees. I was not sure that I was seeing things right, for, where this band of flame was burning I knew there was a small stream, which I would shortly have to cross.

I rode on, watching the fire, which was spreading. The palms and dead branches of over-hanging trees stood outlined against the red flames. The fire spread until it had almost reached the crossing. When I came to the place where I was going to cross the stream, the body of water was aflame. The vines, palms, and pine trees were flaming torches. I could not believe my eyes. I knew that it was impossible for water to burn, yet here I saw the whole stream ablaze.

Waves of flame tossed high to meet and embrace the grasses by the bank and the trees whose branches hung over the water. I watched the fantastic scene until, finally, the flames died down and went out, leaving only the burning trees to convince me that I had not been dreaming. Later I learned that a tank of oil up in the field at Batson Prairie had sprung a leak, and the oil had flowed downstream. A passerby had tossed a lighted cigarette into it, igniting the thick coat of oil on the water and thus producing this rare and beautiful picture.

Occasionally such scenes of beauty or unusual happenings would cross my pathway, resting my mind for a moment from the monotony of gassed people, beaten and injured men, suicide, and accidental death. But when I took time to watch these for a few moments, my conscience nagged me to hurry to some patient who was waiting for me to administer relief.

Not long after Christmas I had two emergencies, I answered the first call immediately. When I arrived at the well where the accident had occurred, I saw a ring of men around the back of a wagon which was loaded with pipe. I noticed that one pipe had been partially pulled out of the wagon and one end of it was resting on the ground. A man sat propped up by the wheel of the wagon, groaning in agony. He was folded up like a jackknife. One of the men told me that the mules had started suddenly, causing the pipe to fall on the man and crush him.

As I straightened him out to see where he was injured, he screamed in agony. I found the right leg broken in two places and that his right shoulder and arm were also broken. As I moved him, I saw blood on his shirt. I set the leg and arm temporarily, instructing the men to make a stretcher to take him to his home. We moved him on the bed. I cut away his shirt to make a more careful examination, and found the right side crushed, with two ribs protruded from the flesh.

I made him as comfortable as possible, and left him, expecting to have a message any moment to write his death certificate. For months he lay, fighting his way back to health. He eventually won out and went back to work.

Finishing this case, I rushed to the second call. I had been informed that a man had been burned, and I naturally thought another boiler had exploded. I learned, instead that the patient had crawled under the boiler to fix some part of it, when the soft plug blew out and let the boiler full of steam down on him. As I could not be immediately reached, another doctor had been called. This other doctor had arrived and, upon seeing the extent of the injuries, he had administered chloroform and left.

When I entered the shack, the patient was still under the influence of the chloroform. I examined him and found the entire upper part of his body cooked. The only unburned flesh above his waist was where his suspenders crossed his back. I had been taught at medical school that when much of the body was burned it meant death. Doubtless the other doctor had been taught the same thing, hence his use of chloroform. When the patient began to come out from under the influence of the chloroform, his suffering was indescribable.

In places only the skin came off. In other places the flesh came off down to the muscle. For months I attended the man daily. When he finally was well, the upper part of his body was a mass of twisted, sunken scars.

The field grew and spread over a wide area, and my practice grew with it. Money was piling up for me, but for some time I realized that I was running a bit of fever. The hard work and drive of the oil fields caused me to know the time was not far distant when I would have to make a change.

STREET SCENES

As I was riding fast to my office from Batson Prairie one afternoon, I heard groans and a call for help. I dismounted and listened. I wrapped the reins around my arm and, leading my horse, walked in the direction of the call. On the ground, near a tree, lay a tall fat man. Groaning loudly, he told me that he had been driving down the road when his horse suddenly became frightened and ran away. The buggy had hit a tree and he had been thrown out and wrapped around one small tree, his leg striking another. As he finished the history of the accident, he closed his eyes and gave a hollow groan. I examined him but could find no broken bones.

Picking up the leg which had struck the tree, I found that the knee cap was broken. I continued to examine and test the leg. Then I told him that the knee cap was broken and the leg was badly bruised, but I thought I could fix him up so the leg would not be stiff in the future. I told him that it would bend now, and was about to go on with my explanations. When I said that his leg would bend, the patient ceased groaning, sat up with a jerk, and yelled, "What did you say?" I nearly dropped his leg, I was so startled. Still yelling at me, he cried, "Don't you fool with that leg if it will bend. That leg's been stiff for twenty years and you let it alone."

Then he told me he had been in an accident twenty years before, had broken his knee cap; that when he got well his leg was stiff; that he had never been able to bend it, and that if it would bend now I was not to touch it. I fixed him up, and along came some men on their way to Saratoga. They took him to the railroad. He went to Beaumont, and I never saw him again.

The next night I went over to chat with the bartender in the saloon next door to my drug store. He was a nice fellow and, when I had a few moments to rest, I often chatted with him. The crowd had not yet come in but, as we were standing there talking, the constable of the town and his deputy entered, both of them intoxicated.

Not wishing to talk with these inebriated officers, the bartender said, "You better go home. The mayor knows you are drunk and is looking for you. If he finds you, he is going to arrest you and lock you up."

We both thought that when the constable heard that he would go home. But it had the opposite effect on him, for he asked the bartender where that damned son-of-a-bitch-mayor was. The bartender told him that the mayor was down the street. In a drunken rage, the officers rushed out to find the mayor.

We were still chatting when in came the mayor of the town, who had also been drinking. He was a short, fat man, with sandy hair and a knobby forehead. His tiny mouse-like ears stood up in the fringe of hair he had left. His wide nose, thick lips, and fat face all had been cooked to a deep red from long years of being soaked in "squirrel whiskey."

We told the mayor that the constable and the deputy were looking for him and were going to arrest him for being drunk. Flying into a tantrum, the mayor rushed out of the door, talking to himself as he went. By this time the bartender and I decided to witness the meeting.

The constable was a tall, thin man, with straggly black hair and moustache. He had a low forehead, a hook nose, long arms, large hands and feet. His mind did not work very fast even when it was not soaked in alcohol. The deputy was just a little scrawny helper, too small to work in the oil field.

We walked to the saloon door just in time to see the constable, deputy and mayor meet in front of my drug store. The constable called the mayor by name and staggered toward him shouting, "In the name of the law I arrest you for being drunk."

The mayor called back, "You long-legged son-of-a-bitch, I refuse arrest."

Making a dash for the mayor, the constable grabbed one of his hands and told his deputy to take hold of the other. In the tussle the three men fell from the sidewalk into the street which was several steps below, piling up on top of each other in a heap. When they tried to untangle themselves in their drunken, limber condition, it was a wild scramble. They began hitting each other, but it was more of a puppet show than a real fight.

Staggering to their feet, the constable and deputy grabbed the mayor's hands again and started down the street with him toward the jail. The exertion of pushing and dragging the fat little mayor soon exhausted the officers. As they stopped, the mayor took advantage of the pause and started back up the street toward my drug store, dragging the constable and deputy with him. Before they could stop the mayor he had pulled them farther back up the street than they had dragged him down. They finally got him stopped and started down the street again to jail. The mayor continued to yell at the top of his voice that he had refused "arrest."

By this time the crowd had gathered and were betting on their favorites as they cheered them on their way to jail. The mayor decided to sit down, but only succeeded in being slid along on his heels. They were all so drunk that they were making very little progress when the constable got a squirrel whiskey idea, which almost knocked off his hat. He called to a man in the crowd and hiccupped, "I deputize you (hic) to take the (hic) hand of the (hic) mayor."

The newly-deputized man entered into the fun heartily and grabbed the mayor's hand. By now the street was full of people and the crowd were about equal divided as to their favorites and were encouraging them, some telling the mayor that he was a "piker" if he went to jail, and others telling the constable to do his duty. By this time the deputy was unable to move from the effects of squirrel whiskey and he called to the constable to deputize someone to take his place. At once the constable deputized another man to take the mayor's hand. The new deputies were only playing along. Resting a bit, the constable went behind the mayor and started to push him to jail, but this also proved a slow march.

By this time the mayor was tired, and he lay down flat in the street. Seized with another whiskey-fueled brainstorm, the constable deputized a man to carry each of the mayor's feet. The constable now took his shoulders, the deputy grabbed him under the hips and, with the crowd cheering, whistling, and yelling, and with the mayor kicking his feet like a fan dancer, they started to jail.

They had gone only a short distance, however, when the new deputies got tired and suddenly turned the mayor loose.

When this was done, the mayor tried to regain his feet, but the constable immediately deputized four other men to take hold of him. With this new help they went about one half block when the recently deputized men became very thirsty and wanted a drink.

The constable immediately fired them and hired a new set who worked a short time, got tired, and quit. Then the constable deputized another set, among whom was the owner of the saloon where the show started. He was a handsome, jolly-looking fellow with several notches on his gun. When the constable deputized the saloon man, he said, "Ah! You go to hell, you son-of-a-bitch."

At this remark those who had been helping dropped the mayor and demanded their pay, which was a round of drinks for helping the state. The constable and deputy found themselves also very thirsty, so they turned the mayor loose and said, "All right, come on." Every one made a rush for the nearest saloon, had their drinks, and came back to take the mayor to jail, but that little dignitary had completely vanished.

Due to the fact that this same mayor had a reputation for slight exaggerations, there was an unwritten law in Saratoga that anyone who repeated what the mayor said must buy drinks for the crowd. When I first came to Saratoga, I did not know the mayor's reputation, and I repeated to a crowd something he had said. Men and women leaped off the high porch where we were all sitting, demanding that I pay up. Realizing what I had done, I bought the drinks. The next time I quoted the mayor I had my fingers crossed and escaped the penalty.

Not long after the unsuccessful attempt to arrest the mayor, I passed a crowd of men on the street. A man seemed to be making a speech. Seeing that he was hilariously drunk, I joined the crowd to see who he was, and recognized the mayor of our town. I went on to my office and, in a short time, he reeled into my drug store. He was yelling and swearing, telling the world how happy he was. He stayed in the store for some time telling me about the earlier days of Saratoga. He had organized a chapter of a popular lodge and I was the medical examiner for it, so we were old "sidekicks." Finally, thirst overcame him and he left.

As the night wore on, he grew more boisterous, ending up by shooting out the lights in the saloon where he was drinking. He was mayor, he said, and by all the legal authority vested in him, he with impunity could, swear, yell, and shoot to his heart's content. Someone took him home toward morning, but he was soon to hear a bit more of his rights of personal liberty.

COURT SCENES

The mayor had a few enemies, some of whom felt that his conduct was beneath the dignity of his exalted office. After several conferences and much debating, they decided that the weighty problem of teaching him deportment fell upon their shoulders. They, therefore, complained to the Kuntz County authorities and started procedure against the noble executive of the town.

The case was set. The mayor and witnesses were summoned. Among the witnesses was a man who had been in the crowd when I had talked with my fingers crossed. This fellow had never recovered from missing that round of drinks for himself and his friends. As we rode up to the trial at Kuntz together, he informed me gleefully that I was to be the first witness, that the judge would ask me what the mayor said, that he and his friends were, in this way, going to get drunk at my expense. I did not reply, but as we rode on I did some thinking.

After we arrived at the courtroom, the judge entered and the bailiff summoned court. I was the first witness called. I took the witness stand after the judge had asked me my name, and the examination started.

In mournful tones the judge inquired of me, "You were in Saratoga on or about a certain night?"

I answered in the affirmative. He then asked me if I had seen the defendant in the case, and if I remembered hearing what he said. I answered, "Yes."

Then he said, "Will the witness kindly repeat what he heard the defendant say?"

The crowd from Saratoga were sitting across from the witness-box, a little to one side of the courtroom. When I started my testimony, they began to stick out their tongues at me making signs of holding glasses in their hands and of drinking deep from a bottle.

I turned a bit in my chair, crossed my legs, dropped my hands in my lap where the Saratoga crowd could see them, took my right hand, pulled the middle finger of my left hand far over the index finger, and pointed to the crossed fingers to focus the Saratoga crowd's eyes on them. Keeping them in that position with my friends looking at them, I told all the defendant did and said that night. I finished and the judge dismissed me.

Another witness was called. Having seen my play, he also crossed his fingers as he testified. Every witness that followed me did the same. The judge, after careful deliberation, decided that the mayor was not disturbing the peace, so we all went home with our money in our pockets, and no one drunk.

A case was tried in front of our court in Saratoga, not long after the mayor's trial. In those days a driller was absolute boss on a rig and took no back-talk from any of his helpers. A few weeks before the above-mentioned case was tried, a boy from the Big Thicket got a job on a rig. This Big Thicket native was very intelligent, in his own estimation, and was not used to the customs of the drillers and the oil field. The driller on the rig spoke to him, one day, in words he did not appreciate, and he told the driller what to do and where to go. Without taking the Big Thicket native's advice, or responding to it, the driller took a Stilson wrench and knocked him out of the derrick. Then he called a couple of rough-necks and told them to take the unconscious native to a shack and send for me.

As soon as the Big Thicket native could walk again, he went down town and complained to the court and had the driller brought into trial. Our mayor, in absence of a judge, took the seat and called the court to order. The old lawyer, who was defending the driller, made an impassioned and flowery speech, and then called the witnesses. All of them were the men helping to drill on this particular rig.

The first witness took the stand and, holding up his right hand, swore to tell the truth and nothing but the truth. In answer to questions about the accident, the witness told solemnly how they were pulling pipe and, from some unknown cause, the derrick seemed to lurch to one side. The plaintiff became scared, as he felt the derrick lurch, and started to run out of it. Without noticing the cross-beams in his fright, he ran blindly against one and struck his head.

The witness was excused and another called. He gave practically the same account of the accident. Witness after witness was called. All the helpers on the rig told the same story. The last witness was just finishing his testimony when a voice from the crowd cried loudly, "Your Honor, I make a motion that the court adjourn and we all go out and get a drink." Immediately almost all in the court yelled, "I second the motion."

Finally the mayor-judge got the crowd quiet, pounding them to order, then he put the motion to a vote. I think every one but the plaintiff and his lawyer roared, "Aye." Before the mayor-judge could adjourn the court, many of the men were out of their seats and running for the door, the mayor-judge closing in fast on the heels of the first one to the door. They all went across the street to the saloon, took several drinks, and returned to take up court. The driller paid for the drinks.

After calling the court to order and before the plaintiff or his lawyer could say a word, the defendant's old lawyer got to his feet and, in an impassioned speech, which fairly brought tears to one's eyes, proved how the plaintiff had falsely accused the defendant of striking him with a wrench. Every eye-witness to the accident had shown how the plaintiff had been injured. The said defendant had shown his helpful and kindly heart, continued the silvery-tongued orator, even under the malicious and untrue accusation which had been offered in the court against him, by offering to pay for drinks for the court, the plaintiff, and his attorney, and all the spectators, thus enabling them to revive their tired minds and bodies and carry on with the case. Therefore, all could testify that the gentle, true, and for giving spirit which the defendant had shown should receive the court's justice. And, furthermore, continued the old lawyer in a sad and injured tone, he prayed the court to see that justice was done and the defendant declared, "Not guilty." Therefore he wished to make a motion to that effect. The motion was received with almost as hearty a response by the spectators as the first one. Without putting the motion to vote, the mayor-judge shouted as best he could, to be heard above the noise, "Defendant declared not guilty." And every one again went out to revive tired minds and bodies at the saloon across the street.

It was in this same place that the county attorney used to come from Kuntz to hold court. He was accustomed to frequenting the gambling houses and, when Lady Luck deserted him and he would lose his bank roll at poker or some other game, he would come to Saratoga and hold court. He was always sure of retrieving his losses from the fines which he took in from the pimps and the prostitutes. Each time, before he appeared, he would send a deputy sheriff down and round up this class of people in herds, and bring them into court so that he could fine them for "vagrancy."

He would open the cases by asking the accused their names and then go into a long discussion about the fact that the accused did not have any visible means of support, and would end by asking them to show evidences of such means of support. Of course, the pimps and ladies could not show any such evidence, so he would say, "You are fined twenty-five dollars and costs. Next case please."

When he would finish fining and collecting from these two classes, he would not need to hold court for some time. The underworld characters hated him intensely, but they had no redress and could do nothing except to pay the fines that he had levied against them.

One day, when he was holding court in Saratoga, he had finished fining all the pimps and had started on the cases against the girls. Calling the first case, he asked the shy violet to give her name. She was a cute little girl about fifty years old, not over five feet tall, and weighing about two hundred pounds, as broad as she was tall. With large ears, which had the appearance of leaning forward, small brown crossed eyes, and triple chin below a wide mouth filled with dirty buck teeth, she would never have been a candidate for the queen in a Miss America beauty contest.

The county attorney was more than half drunk when he began court, and a few swigs from a bottle of "white mule" during intermission had not been any aid him in finding sobriety. His pockets were bulging from the fines he had already collected, and the world looked good to him; so he felt some what inclined to be magnanimous. Deciding to lighten the dreariness of the court procedure a bit, he became a bit playful with the little girl he was trying. He went through with his regular routine, but he chose to add many humorous extras thrown in. Then he asked the dainty kitten in front of him whether or not she had any visible means of support.

She dropped her head and shyly said, "Yes."

The county attorney was too drunk to catch the hate in her voice.

"Very well, will you please show the court the means of your support," he commanded, "or pay a fine of twenty-five dollars and costs."

She did not hesitate. Bending forward from her hips as if she were making a bow to the county attorney, and taking hold of the bottom of her skirts with both hands, she started to straighten up. By that time the judge was yelling, "Not guilty! Put down your dress! Not guilty!"

Pandemonium broke out in the court room at the evidence of the visible means of support, and the judge shouted, "Court adjourned!"

The spectators roared with laughter and, grabbing the county attorney, rushed him toward the saloon.

"This time you buy drinks for the town," they demanded, and called to the pimps, girls, gamblers, and those in the street to come and drink on the law. When they were through, the drinks had cost the county attorney so much he was ready to hold court again.

I had seen life in all its phases in the oil field, so I thought, but the thing that made me decide to change my location and go some place where I could at least, be buried in decency and order, was a funeral service for one of the Saratoga prostitutes. The pimps, gamblers, saloon-men and girls were her mourners. When they lowered her coffin into the grave and covered it up, the question arose among them as to an appropriate service.

Many of those standing around the grave had come in contact with some kind of Christian training in their younger days. All of them believed that there was a Hereafter. They, therefore, felt that some kind of a service should be held at the grave. But what kind? None of them could pray. Sin had blotted out all desire for and remembrance of prayer. After conferring for a few minutes, they finally decided that maybe they should sing something. But no one knew a hymn. Again they went into a huddle.

Finally, one old drunk, after very deep thought, exclaimed, "I've got it! We will sing the new song which has just come out."

Every one clapped him on the back and told him that he was a genius. Tuning up in his whiskey-soaked voice, he led the throng in singing:

> "We were born into this world,
> All naked and bare.
> We go through it with sorrow and care;
> When we die we are going no one knows where,
> But if we are rounders here,
> We will be rounders there."

CPSIA information can be obtained
at www.ICGtesting.com
Printed in the USA
BVHW082223221219
567537BV00002B/12/P